Faith-FULL and Fit

The Christian's Guide to Becoming Spiritually and Physically Fit

"So whether you eat or drink, or whatever you do, do it all for the glory of God."
(1 Corinthians 10:31)

CARLA T. HARDY, MS, CSCS

WESTBOW
PRESS®
A DIVISION OF THOMAS NELSON
& ZONDERVAN

WestBow Press books may be ordered through booksellers or by contacting:

WestBow Press
A Division of Thomas Nelson & Zondervan
1663 Liberty Drive
Bloomington, IN 47403
www.westbowpress.com
1 (866) 928-1240

ISBN: 978-1-4908-8994-8 (sc)
ISBN: 978-1-4908-8996-2 (hc)
ISBN: 978-1-4908-8995-5 (e)

Library of Congress Control Number: 2015920507

Print information available on the last page.

WestBow Press rev. date: 01/05/2016

Table of Contents

―――――――∽――――――

INTRODUCTION

GET STARTED!!

NUTRITION: FEED THE SPIRIT INSTEAD

FITNESS

FAITH

To my mother—gone but not forgotten. You are the woman I aspire to be and the love that I will always miss. Thank you so much for loving me despite my flaws. Although you are not here physically to read this in person, I know you see.

Acknowledgements

———∽———

I would like to thank all those who had a hand in helping me reach this pivotal point in my journey. Everyone in my life in some way helped mold me and push me to reach further. Whether by your teachings, love, smiles, encouragement or rejections, you are greatly appreciated.

Special thanks to all my family, especially my father, sisters and brother. Thank you to my friends who have supported me throughout my endeavors. To my Pastor, Mark A. Couch and First Lady Ivy Coach, your faith in me has been a guiding light in pushing me further towards my kingdom purpose. To the ladies of Faith for Fitness, thanks so much for allowing me to be a part of your world. Working with you all has been a God-send.

All Scriptures have been taken from the New International Version of the Bible, unless otherwise indicated.

Preface

—◊—

Do you not know that your body is a temple of the Holy Spirit, who is in you, whom you have received from God? You are not your own; you were bought at a price. Therefore honor God with your body.

1 Corinthians 6:19–20

Introduction

———⌒⌒———

Nourishing your body . . .
Feeding your Soul . . .

Becoming Faith-Full And Fit

———— ✦ ————

If somebody offered you the keys to add 10 years to your existence, improve your quality of life, well being and spiritual health; would you take them and use them? The knowledge you gain within *Faith-FULL and Fit* will give you those keys. All you have to do is use them—place them in the lock and turn . . . .

There is a direct relationship between faith/spirituality and health. God made us with a soul and body and they work together in an amazing way. *Faith-FULL and Fit* was created to instruct individuals on the basics of fitness, wellness and healthy living based on Christian principles and the Word of God. This book will equip you with the knowledge to become wiser in your nutritional choices, improve your fitness, strengthen your faith and grow closer to God. Many books, fad diets and exercise programs give you the physical tools to get healthy, but most of them do not offer a method to change the way you think, or a means to change your heart and spirit. All of those components combined lead our actions and daily living habits.

Because the soul and body are so closely intertwined, it is nearly impossible to heal the body without healing the soul. They must work together for you to reach full health and happiness. One without the other is simply inadequate. To have a healthy body, we must have a healthy spirit also.

We pray and ask God to help guide us in every other aspect of our lives: family, marriage, fears, sickness, etc. Why not health and fitness?

You do not have, because you do not ask God (James 4:2).
Prayer is key.

Then you will call upon me and come and pray to me, and I will listen to you (Jeremiah 29:12)

Pray and ask God for the change in your life you wish to see. Ask for a changed heart and mind, changed actions and habits . . . And a permanent change at that. "To pray is to change," writes Richard Foster in Celebration of Discipline. "Prayer is the central avenue God uses to transform us." This is where all of your life changing commitments should start, with prayer and seeking God. No journey is safe to take without God.

Never will I leave you; never will I forsake you (Hebrews 13:5)

Use the prayers found here in *Faith-FULL and Fit* or create your own. He is with you through it all.

We struggle every day with fighting our urges, temptations, etc. But many times our battles are not truly physical, but in our spiritual deprivations. However, we use vices of the flesh (food, people, etc.) to fill the voids we are lacking in our spiritual lives.

Faith-FULL and Fit uses an introspective approach to improving your lifestyle where you look within first, healing the body from the inside out. It will teach you to recognize, focus on and change the inner/spiritual issues first. Inward cleansing and healing will in turn produce an outward change. You will develop a closer relationship with God and learn to let him lead, all while renewing your heart and mind to elicit lasting, healthier decisions. This book will not only give you the physical tools you need to live a healthy lifestyle and maintain it, but more importantly, it will also offer you biblical and spiritual guidance to help you fill the hollowness in your spirit that causes you to seek physical fulfillment. What God promises us through prayer, his Word and our faith in him cannot be matched by any worldly remedy.

. . . and by his wounds we are healed (Isaiah 53:5)

It is my hope that the resources in *Faith-FULL and Fit* will help you grow knowledgeable about fitness, nutrition and overall wellness. Allow you to put an end to the yo-yo dieting, emotional eating and lack of motivation. As well as impart the means to grow stronger in your faith and in the Word of God.

True Healing

———— ⌒⌒ ————

Often, the only true hope for healing from affliction, deliverance from bad habits, and restoration from sin is through divine intervention. If not for God giving us strength, we would not get out of the ruts or the valleys in which we find ourselves. We must be willing to call on the name of Jesus in order to allow him to come in and intervene on our behalf, so that we can experience divine healing.

If you are reading Faith-FULL and Fit, you are probably fed up with the way you were doing things month after month and year after year, constantly dealing with the same afflictions, weight problems or depression. These situations are just a few of the tactics Satan uses to **"steal, kill and destroy" (John 10:10)** the fruit of our lives and ultimately us. If the enemy can keep us in the same holding pattern, then we will never take flight and reach our destinations or our destiny in Christ!

But we can rejoice, because at some point, you realized that you were not living your best, and that God intends so much more for you. In your quiet hour you cried out:

"Heal me O lord, and I will be healed; Save me, and I will be saved, for you are the one I praise" (Jeremiah 17:14).

As you embark on this total body, mind and spirit makeover, you are going to laugh at times and cry at others. Anything worth having is worth working for, and there will be plenty of days when it will seem impossible. You may grow tired and frustrated, but it is during these moments of weakness that you must get in the Word; lean on God and be encouraged

Remember: you are a work in progress and God has not given up on you, so you cannot give up on yourself. It is through his strength that you overcome. God's promises are platforms on which you can and must stand!

"God is not a man, that he should lie" (Numbers 23:19)
So when he says . . .

"But I will restore you to health and heal your wounds, declares the LORD . . ." (Jeremiah 30:17)
. . . know that it is done.

What the world means for your down fall, God will ultimately work out for your good. The health and healing you are praying for will be restored, and you will rejoice.

"Behold, I will bring it health and healing; I will heal them and reveal to them the abundance of peace and truth" (Jeremiah 33:6).

I thank God for your obedience and for your efforts. We only get one go at this journey called life; there is no dress rehearsal and no second take. I applaud your dedication to yourself, your family and most importantly, to God.

Finding And Filling Life's Voids

———— ❧ ————

The *Faith-FULL and Fit* journey to improved health and wellness requires more than just changing your nutritional and exercise habits. To elicit a permanent change in your life, you must change the underlying cause of your actions. That means delving into the reasons you do the things you do, discovering what your issues are and finding solutions to resolve them.

Many times we run away from our problems or use worldly things to smother the ill feelings that are plaguing us. We find comfort in food, alcohol, sex, drugs, etc. They allow us to forget our troubles, even if it is only temporary. Some of us may find ourselves constantly resorting to these methods, so much so that they become habits or addictions that never allow us to address and work out the real cause of our problems. This is because they are always masked by this temporary worldly "high".

Have you ever asked yourself why you make detrimental decisions? "Why do I eat when I'm not hungry?" "Why do I drink so much?" "Why do I always have to be involved with someone, even if it is not a healthy relationship for me?" "Why is my self-esteem so low?" "Why can't I find true happiness in anyone or anything?" For most, the answer is simple: you have lost your connection with God. What we do not realize is that the world's happiness is temporary, but God's joy is forever and your true happiness lies within him. If you know that God will supply all your needs, then there is no need to use these worldly devices to suppress your pain, mask your problems and give you comfort.

And my God will meet all your needs according to his glorious riches in Christ Jesus (Philippians 4:19)

Replace your vices with God's love and his Word.

To begin filling the voids in your life, you must first figure out where you lack. As long as you are using the world's comforts to mask your issues, you will never figure them out. This is because we use these attachments to help us forget about our problems and push them as far back in our subconscious as possible. How can you possibly deal with the real issue if it is always suppressed? Though bringing your issues to the forefront may hurt, it is a necessary evil to move forward.

It was not until Sunday, October 3rd, 2010 during church service that I was able to see that I too was using the resources and people around me to help me cope with my problems instead of dealing with them. I had awakened in a melancholy mood for no reason at all. Nothing drastic had changed, but I was feeling pretty low, lonely and lost. The one thing I remember vividly is the choir singing *Take Back What the Devil Stole From Me* and the pastor changing his sermon because he had been led by the Spirit to do so. God must have known I needed to hear a message that spoke directly to me. I had no idea I was so lost in my own world. I cried during the entire sermon and through communion. I cannot tell you the exact words of the sermon that day, but I can tell you what thoughts it conjured up. I had let the devil steal my joy and I had to take it back.

Your enemy the devil prowls around like a roaring lion looking for someone to devour (1 Peter 5:8)

I relied on food, people and money to bring me so-called "happiness." Somehow, I had let the world decide for me what things should bring me joy. I was so enthralled with providing my own happiness—without God—that I depleted all of my savings. I spent it all, not to pay necessary bills, like the mortgage, lights, gas, etc., but to try and satisfy the emptiness inside me with material things. Instead, I created unnecessary debt trying to please myself and attain the world's definition of "happiness."

I spent money on clothes, shoes and friends, and I cannot account for most of it. I spent years and many dollars trying to fix my body so it would be physically pleasing to man. I exhausted many hours on exercise and yo-yo dieting. I was so caught up in what people thought of my appearance, seeking worldly gratification and man's love, that I would not even cut my hair because everyone else liked it longer. My focus was all wrong. I was a people pleaser. I did great deeds, but my focus was to please man and not God. Sometimes it would even hurt me if I was unable to satisfy the people around me. In my mind, if I could please them, they would stay, love me and I would not be lonely. I incessantly reached out to man to fill and complete me and always came back empty handed.

How did I get there? My search for love began in 2000 when I was 21. That year, I lost my mother. The hollowness I felt within me was like a black abyss of pain, sorrow and confusion. My mother's love was like no other. She would go without just so I could have and loved me despite my flaws. She gave me a love that has never been matched in my life. When she passed, that love was gone. I was lost and began searching (unconsciously) for the love that had been taken from me. Love. That is what I wanted. That is what I needed.

I dated for years, never fully attaching myself emotionally to anyone. I would linger in relationships where I did not have to commit and give my all, just so I would not have to feel the hurt I felt when I lost my mother. The cycle of dating men I knew that I could never fully be with, commit to and have them commit to me, had become so monotonous it was almost insane. Insanity—doing the same thing over and over and expecting different results. It took me years before I even realized what I was doing or, more importantly, why I was doing it. Although I thought I was ready for love, I was very guarded and not equipped to love anyone.

The harder I tried to find love, the lonelier I felt, because all my attempts failed. The key word here is "my". I did what "I" thought would bring love in my life. I had stepped into a few relationships without letting God lead me, and they left me with wounds deeper than any ocean. Those wounds kept me from letting go and truly loving someone else and letting someone else love me. To be loved, to feel love, to give love was what I desired most but it eluded me. Love was also the one thing I would not allow in my life for fear of being hurt again.

I knew being and feeling lonely was my biggest issue. I was lonely even though I had plenty of family and friends surrounding me. Lonely even though I knew God was always with me. At least I thought I knew. It took a lot of soul searching for me to realize that my inner loneliness and quest to be loved was driving many of my detrimental actions. Because I had been suppressing my pain and comforting myself through the flesh, I didn't realize my issues lay in my disconnected spirit. An empty, longing spirit that was disconnected from God's love was the underlying cause that fueled many of my decisions. Instead of dealing with my issues head on, I sought comfort in food, material possessions and man, drowning my pain in the world's temporary remedies.

I was trying to fill my voids in the world, but the love I sought, I had all along. It was in God.

. . . God is love (1 John 4:8)

Loneliness and seeking love may not be your void. But to figure it out, you will have to eliminate the distractions in your life so you can understand what your void is. You cannot find a solution to a problem until you figure out what the problem is. Prayerfully ask God to remove those vices on which you depend to camouflage your issues and stand on his Word. Allow yourself to depend on God for comfort.

Now my eyes will be open and my ears attentive to the prayers offered in this place (2 Chronicles 7:15)

Once you have figured out what your void is, fill your emptiness by finding your purpose in God's kingdom. Either we live to please ourselves, or we live to please God. Live to please God. We please God when we live by faith and by his Word. Pleasing God results in our everlasting joy.

If My people, who are called by My name, shall humble themselves and pray, and seek My face, and turn from their wicked ways, then I will hear from Heaven and will forgive their sin and will heal their land (2 Chronicles 7:14)

Permanent transformation works from the inside out, healing the spirit and changing the mind. Once you have dealt with the inner issues that have been plaguing you, you can step forward into a changed action plan. Because you have healed the spirit, by changing your heart and mind, new actions and new habits are sure to follow.

See the former things have taken place, and new things I declare; before they spring into being I announce them to you. (Isaiah 42:13)

Prayer

———⌁———

Lord, I humbly come to you asking you to guide me in your way.
I ask that you strip me of those things that are not of your will and
those that keep me blinded from my purpose in your kingdom.
Lord, open my heart so that I may accept your love and know that
you will never leave nor forsake me.
Open my mind so that I may see my problems.
Right now Lord, I am ready to look at whatever truth you
want to reveal to me.
Help me deal with them so I can move forward.
Heal my spirit and fill any and all voids in my life with your love.
I know there may be pain during this process,
but true happiness awaits.
I desire an everlasting change in my life.
Please strengthen my faith so I can stand on your Word.
Show me my purpose, so I can fulfill your will Lord
and be a blessing.
Thank You for filling my spirit with your unconditional love.
In Jesus' name I pray,

AMEN

Get Started!!

---ᴏᴠᴑ---

How long will you lie there you sluggard? When will you get up from your sleep?
Proverbs 6:9

Getting Started

———— ⌒∽ ————

You are now ready to get started and step into your new health and fitness action plan. As you start your new journey, know that God is with you. Don't be afraid, he will be with you on this journey as with all others.

No one will be able to stand up against you all the days of your life. As I was with Moses, so I will be with you; I will never leave you nor forsake you. (Joshua 1:5).

Your spirit and longings are being fulfilled, so let's take action. But before you step into your plan, evaluate whether your heart and mind are in the right place. Begin by asking yourself, "What are my reasons for wanting to live a healthier lifestyle?" Is it to preserve God's temple?

"Don't you realize that your body is the temple of the Holy Spirit, who lives in you and was given to you by God? You do not belong to yourself, for God bought you with a high price. So you must honor God with your body" (Corinthians 6:19-20).

Is it to improve your health? Or is it for a better body? Are you motived by vanity? Pride in your appearance should not overshadow your desire to honor God.

Getting healthy for vain reasons is meaningless and pointless.

Meaningless! Meaningless! Says the teacher. Utterly meaningless. Everything is meaningless (Ecclesiastes 1:2).

If there is no purpose behind your actions, then what are you doing it for?

Yet when I surveyed all that my hands had done and I toiled to achieve, everything was meaningless, a chasing wind; nothing was gained under the sun (Ecclesiastes 1:11)

You do not want your hard-work and toil to be for nothing. When your purpose in getting healthy is to bless God's kingdom, your struggles to reach your goals become lighter. God will bless and guide what is done to please him. Therefore, having your heart and mind in the right place when you start your program is a must. Figure out what a "healthier you" can offer as a blessing and let that be your motivation to achieve optimal wellness.

As he thinketh in his heart, so he is (Proverbs 23:7).

Finally, brothers, whatever is true, whatever is noble, whatever is right, whatever is pure, whatever is lovely, whatever is admirable—if anything is excellent or praiseworthy—think about such things (Philippians 4:8)

Start your health and fitness journey with God—let God lead! Sometimes we try to go ahead of God and fail. If you have already begun, back up and allow God to go first. Do not pray and ask God for guidance then go out and try to do it on your own. Going about it your own way is the wrong way. Before you move, hear from God and he will guide you to the path which you are to take.

Are you so foolish? After beginning with the Spirit, you are now trying to attain your goal by human effort (Galatians 3:3)

If you let God lead, he will begin his work within you. You are a beautiful work in progress. Once God begins, he will not stop until it is done.

I am confident of this, that he who began a good work in you will carry it out on to completion until the day of Christ Jesus (Philippians 1:6).

The Lord has plans for you . . .

For I know the plans I have for you, declares the Lord, plans to prosper you and not harm you, plans to give you hope for a future (Jeremiah 29:11)

You have to be willing to go through the process to receive your good measure and your new thing—the process of slowly improving your nutritional habits, exercise habits and increasing your faith in God. All of it done to better yourself, so you can be used as a blessing to God's kingdom. Know that through your process, your blessings are coming. Remember, you have to be blessed to bless someone else.

. . . It is more blessed to give than to receive (Acts 20:35)

When you are beginning to walk into change, whatever it may be in life, focus on fixing the problem and not the results. For example, you may want to lose weight. You should concentrate on changing your nutritional and exercise habits instead of your weight loss. If you fix the problem, the results will come. Do not sabotage yourself from the start because your focus is wrong. Make changes that will aid you in doing the will of God, instead of making changes for selfish purposes. Seek God first in your journey and make sure your desire for a particular change is within his will.

Now that your heart and mind are in the right place, eliminate the excuses. If you really want to make changes in your life, you do not need anyone but God. "Such and such said they were going to help me, so I did not do it." You do not have to wait on anyone but God to get started on your journey. Stop trying to justify not beginning and just do it. You cannot move forward until you let go of your excuses and embrace where God is leading you.

Forget the former things; do not dwell on the past. See I am doing a new thing! (Isaiah 43:18-19).

Forget your past excuses, failures and setbacks. You can never grab onto the next vine and swing forward if you are afraid to let go of the vine you are holding on to. You will just be stuck in the middle going nowhere. Let go and use those former things as your springboard to catapult you into this new God-led excursion.

Out of all that you want and desire from this world, renewed health or other, NEVER FORGET GOD!

Prayer

———❧———

Lord, I am embarking on a new journey, and I need you now, as I
always have.
I pray for power, strength and self-love to keep me motivated and
moving forward in a positive direction.
Lord, change my heart, my mind, my spirit and my actions so they
are in line with your will for me.
Feed my spirit with your love and satisfy me with your Word.
Lead me so I that may be a blessing to your kingdom.
You are my bread of life.
Today I am placing it all in your hands.
Guide me in your way and use me as you see fit.

AMEN

Taking Steps

———— ⌀ ————

Now that your soul-tending is progressing, taking steps to a permanently healthier you is next. Do not just hop onto the next fad diet or "gimmick" exercise program. Take the time to research what is going to work best for you and help you reach your desired goals.

A simple man believes anything, but a prudent man gives thought to his steps." (Proverbs 14:15).

Ask the Lord to guide your steps, for He will never lead you in the wrong direction.

Start your *Faith-FULL and Fit* journey by making a promise to yourself, your loved ones and God that you will see your endeavors through to completion. At the end of this chapter, you will find a commitment contract. Fill this out as a pledge to yourself to become healthier. Hold yourself accountable for your actions.

Consult your physician to ensure you are healthy enough to begin an exercise program. Also inquire about any suggestions he can offer concerning any limitations you should consider when choosing an exercise and nutrition plan that is right for you. Have your physician or fitness professional evaluate your physical fitness levels before you get started. These measurements will provide you with valuable information to base your goals on, determine what level/intensity your fitness plan should begin with and allow you to see where you are versus where you should be.

On the subsequent pages, you will learn the importance of knowing your physical fitness numbers and guidelines to setting realistic goals that will keep you motivated.

FAITH-FULL AND FIT COMMITMENT CONTRACT

Today, I _____, am making
a commitment to myself to live healthier, be wiser in my lifestyle
choices and stronger in my faith. I am willing to put in the work
necessary to manifest the desired results and improve my mental,
physical, emotional and spiritual well-being. I understand that living
healthfully is a lifetime change, there is no quick fix and giving up
is not an option. I will see this through to completion. I understand
that for me to reach my goals, I must work hard, be open to change
and consistent in my efforts. I am determined and will use the
information found in *Faith-FULL and Fit* to help guide me to a
healthier way of life.

By signing below, I am committed to improving my overall health
and committed to changing my lifestyle to elicit the results I desire.

Signature: _____ Date: _____

My father used to make me recite:

**"If a task is once begun, never leave it
until its done. Whether the work great
or small, do it well or not at all."**

*" . . . faith by itself, if it is not accompanied by action,
is dead." (James 2:17)*

Knowing Your Numbers

———— ∞ ————

Knowing your fitness numbers gives you a baseline of where you are physically, as well as a point to start tracking your progress. Your initial fitness assessment will show what areas need improvement to reach optimal health. Your basic fitness assessment should include tests for cardio-respiratory fitness, muscular strength and endurance, body composition and flexibility. Other tests will provide even more detailed information.

Cardio-respiratory Fitness—The ability of large muscles to perform dynamic, moderate-to-high intensity exercise for prolonged periods.

Muscular Strength—The maximal force that can be generated by a specific muscle or muscle group.

Muscular Endurance—The ability of a muscle or muscle group to execute repeated contractions over a period of time.

Body Composition—The relative percentage of body weight that is fat and fat-free tissue. It is the percentage of the body that is fat versus lean mass (which includes muscles, bones and organs).

Flexibility—The ability to move a joint through its complete range of motion.

Blood Pressure—Refers to two different pressures in the blood vessels. Systolic pressure is the pressure in the vessels when the heart contracts and the diastolic pressure is represented when the heart is in full relaxation. This number is significant because if it is high for a prolonged period of time, it can be an indicator of other disease states and can cause malfunctions in the body, such as damaged blood vessels, kidneys, brain and heart.

Heart Rate—The number of times the heart beats per minute.

Another important baseline measure is your resting metabolic rate, or RMR. When you hear people talk about your metabolism, this is the number they are referring to. RMR represents how many calories you would burn at absolute rest, as in sleeping for 24 hours straight. This baseline number is the number of calories the body would require to maintain your current weight. For example: If Lee has an RMR of 2000 calories, he would need to consume 2000 calories to keep his weight the same. If Lee consumed less than 2000 calories, he would begin to see his weight decrease. If he consumed more than 2000 calories per day, he would eventually gain weight.

If you are unable to complete a full fitness assessment, establishing and knowing your weight and RMR (resting metabolic rate) will be very useful in reaching your fitness goals. We will go into more detail about RMR in the nutrition section of *Faith-FULL and Fit*, ESTABLISHING YOUR RMR.

Body Composition

—— ∽ ——

There are several ways to measure body composition or body fatness. The Body Mass Index (BMI) scale is a ratio of one's weight to height. BMI is most often used to assess body composition, but has its limitations. Be mindful that this scale does not take into consideration one's muscularity, and can be highly inaccurate for a muscular individual. According to the BMI chart, a body builder would most likely be obese, although they may only have a small percentage of body fat. Therefore, a scale that measures your body fat percentage is more relevant.

Body fat percentage can be measured in several ways; 3- or 7 Site skin-fold using calipers, bioelectrical impedance and hydrostatic weighing are some of the tools. Hydrostatic weighing is the gold standard, but is the least available.

Following are the ranked scales for BMI (Body mass index) and body fat percentage. Get your measurements taken and see where you fall. Do you need improvement? Or should you maintain?

(BMI) = Weight (kg) divided by Height (m) squared.

BMI (kg/m2)

Underweight" <18.5
Normal" 18.5 - 24.9
Overweight" 25.0 - 29.9
Obese Class I" 30.0 - 34.9
Obese Class II" 35.0 - 39.9
Obese Class III" > or equal to 40

Provided by the American College of Sports Medicine

Getting your body fat percentage measured is a much better method of defining your body composition. This scale describes the ratio of lean mass (muscles, bones, organs) to fat mass in the body.

Body Fat Classifications

	Men	Women
Unhealthy Low (Not recommended)	<5%	<12%
Elite Athlete	5-7%	12-14%
Excellent	8-10%	15-18%
Good	11-19%	18-25%
Borderline	19-24%	26-31%
Unhealthy High	>24%	>32%

Blood Pressure Classifications for Adult Aged 18 Years and Older		
Category	Systolic Blood Pressure (mmHg)	Diastolic Pressure (mmHg)
Optimal	< 120 and	< 80
Normal	120 -129 and	80 - 84
High Normal	130 -139 or	85 - 89
Hypertension		
Stage 1	140 - 159 or	90 - 99
Stage 2	150 - 179 or	100 - 109
Stage 3	≥ 180 or	≥ 110

* Taken from American College of Sports Medicine. ACSM's Guidelines for Exercise Testing and Prescription. 6th ed., pg. 41-42. Baltimore, MD: American College of Sprots Medicine, 2000.

Setting Goals

———— ✑ ————

You are geared up and ready to go, and already know what you want to accomplish. But are your expectations reasonable? Goals should be realistic and tangible. Setting goals that are unrealistic can negatively affect your program and also discourage you. Make sure your goals are also measureable. Do not just say I want to lose weight; put a number and date to it. "I want to lose 8lb in the next 30 days." Set both health-related and spiritual goals. Using the following criteria when setting your goals and you will be well on your way.

Set Realistic Goals

By telling yourself that you are going to look like Halle Berry or Terrill Owens, or that you are going to break the 100m sprint world record is most likely setting you up for failure. On the other hand, if you plan to lose one pound a week by exercising 3 times a week for at least 30 minutes, along with following a healthy nutritional plan, you are setting a realistic and attainable goal for yourself.

Set Mini Goals

Perhaps one reason you have not reached your past goals is because the goal you set was too much to accomplish at one time. Setting mini goals will help you reach your overall objective in steps, whether it be to lose weight or improve your cardiovascular fitness. For instance, if your aspiration is to lose 50 pounds, begin by focusing on losing 10 pounds. Before you know it, you will have hit your mark.

Find a Support System

Find an exercise partner as a "buddy" support system to help you stay accountable. Having this accountability will allow you to reach your target much easier versus going at it alone. You can encourage each other and can help each other when you find yourself making excuses, such as "I'm too tired," or, "It's too late, so I will double my time tomorrow." Of course, tomorrow never comes.

Two are better than one . . . . If one falls down, his friend can help him up (Ecclesiastes 4:9–10).

Constructively Deal with Setbacks

Everyone will slip up every now and then. Deal with it by thinking positively. Do not allow it to hinder your overall goal. Maybe there were unpreventable circumstances that halted your progress. Think of it only as a detour and get back on track the next day. Feeling guilty for hitting a stumbling block will not help you, so shake it off and move forward. Tomorrow is a new day and a new beginning. An occasional miss or slip up will not derail your overall goal, but make those deviations a rare occurrence.

Forget the former things; do not dwell on the past . . ." (Isaiah 43:18–19).

Reward Yourself

Yes, you can reward yourself. You can do so each time you surpass your mini goal! But avoid treating yourself with items or activities that can adversely affect your accomplishments, such as chocolate or high calorie meals. Instead, try a sassy new dress or buy those "Oh So Sweet" shoes you have been eyeing! Rewarding yourself allows you to enjoy your successes and keeps you motivated. Positive reinforcement produces positive results.

Create Spiritual Goals

What are some things you need to change in your spiritual life? Sit down and evaluate what areas need work and add them to your list of goals. You may reach all of the external/outward goals you have set for yourself, but if your spirit is empty you have not succeeded. An increased spirit is by far the most important goal you can obtain. "Smaller body, larger spirit." The best results work from the inside out.

Use the next page, to write out your short-term, mid-term and long-term goals. You should aspire to achieve short-term goals within the next 12 weeks, mid-term goals in the next 3-6 months, and long-term goals in the next 6-12 months or longer.

MY GOALS

Choose three short-term goals you would like to accomplish in the next 12 weeks.

1. _____
2. _____
3. _____

Choose three mid-term goals you would like to accomplish in the next 3-6 months.

1. _____
2. _____
3. _____

Choose three long term goals that you would like to accomplish in the next six months to one year and beyond.

1. _____
2. _____
3. _____

Choose three spiritual goals you would like to accomplish.

1. _____

2. _____

3. _____

Nutrition:
Feed the Spirit Instead

———— ✑ ————

You satisfy me more than the richest of foods. Psalm 63:5 (NLT)

Therefore, fill your spirit and not your belly . . . .

Nutrition Basics

———— ✂ ————

Improving your nutritional habits can be a daunting task. We become bogged down with so much information that we are at a loss as where to start. You may find yourself asking; "What should I eat? What foods are right for me? How many calories do I need?" The list goes on and on.

The truth is, there is no single answer to this question because everyone is different. We have different body types, health/nutritional concerns, activity levels and foods we prefer.

The most important aspect of a healthy nutritional plan is making sure it fits into your life and it is maintainable. All the diets you have tried in the past were not sustainable; otherwise you would still be on them.

Today, we will banish the word "diet" completely. It insinuates that something is being taken away, and that is not the case at all. What we are actually doing is enhancing—enhancing the nutritive value of the foods we choose to eat and enhancing our knowledge about what foods are best to fuel our bodies.

In the nutrition section of *Faith-FULL and Fit*, you will learn what role food should play in your life and how the way we "view" food dictates why and how much we eat. You will also acquire the knowledge base to choose healthier foods and make basic modifications to your nutritional plan to help you achieve your health and wellness goals.

There are so many "diet" plans out there, it would take years to research them all. But remember, we have banished the word "diet" from our vocabulary, so we will not need those anyway. What we intend to do is make small changes over time to create a flavorful nutrition plan that can be maintained for a lifetime. Small changes yield big results. Changing your nutritional habits will not happen overnight.

But over time and with consistent practice, eating healthfully will become second nature. Practice makes perfect.

Where should you begin? Start here with these seven rules of thumb. These few tips should become the foundation for your nutritional plan.

Eat Plenty of Vegetables—Eat a variety of vegetables—the more colorful, the better. Different vegetables provide different nutrients. Therefore, choosing a variety will ensure the body gets an adequate amount of nutrients. Eat at least 5 servings of vegetables per day.

Please test your servants for ten days: Give us nothing but vegetables to eat and water to drink. Then compare our appearance with that of the young men who eat the royal food ... (Daniel 1:12-13)

At the end of the ten days they looked healthier and better nourished than any of the young men who ate the royal food (Daniel 1:15)

Get Your Fix of Fruit—Eat a variety of fruit. Choose fresh, frozen or canned (in juice), even dried fruit in small amounts. Aim for 2-3 servings per day.

Choose Complex Carbohydrates—Choose whole grain breads, cereals, Brown rice, etc. Complex carbohydrates are higher in fiber and other nutrients than refined grains, which have been stripped of those components during processing.

Love Lean Protein—Choose lean meats, poultry and fish—lean protein has less fat and less calories. Vegetarian protein sources include beans, nuts, peas and seeds.

Know Your Fats—Generally speaking, your fat intake should be less than 30% of your day's calories. Look for foods low in saturated fat, trans-fat and cholesterol.

Limit Your Sugar and Salt Intake—Beware of sugary foods and beverages that offer plenty of empty calories, without any nutritive value. Also look out for salty foods, which can increase blood pressure and negatively affect the kidneys and heart if too much is consumed over a long period of time.

Be Mindful of Portion Sizes—Most times, our portion sizes are too large, often doubling or even tripling the actual calories we think we are consuming. Use your *Faith-FULL and Fit* Portion Size Guide as a reference.

Starting a new and different nutritional plan can be difficult. So think of these two words when you start: SIMPLE and SLOW. Simplify in the beginning and build up a strong foundation. Take it slow; your new eating habits will take time to establish.

Simplify. It can be hard to count calories and measure your portions. If so, think of your nutrition plan in terms of variety and color. Choose healthy foods you know you love and incorporate new food items gradually. As you continue, your eating will become healthier and more delicious.

Start slowly and make changes to your eating habits over time. Trying to change everything in your nutrition plan at one time is not realistic and can halt your progress. You can lose motivation because you are unable to maintain the unrealistic expectations you have set for yourself. You will find yourself cheating and eventually give up completely if you do not step into your changes gradually. Take small steps, like adding more water if you are not drinking enough or gradually decreasing the amount of food you eat until you are eating a regular portion size. As your small changes become habit, you can continue to add more healthy choices to your plan.

If taking the necessary steps to start a new nutritional program is not possible for you right now, do not fret. There are a few small changes you can make now that will give great results.

Daily Tips: What Can I Do Right Now That Will Make a Difference?

1. Drink plenty of water. Consume at least half your body weight in ounces.
   Example: If Anne is 100 pounds, she should drink 50 ounces or more of water per day. This is approximately eight 8-ounce glasses per day.
2. Drink a glass of water 20 minutes prior to meal time to alert the brain that you are beginning to eat. This may aid you in feeling satisfied (full) sooner.
3. Drink ½ the amount of caloric beverages (soda, juice, etc.) you usually drink per day.
4. Eat a vegetarian meal at least 3 times per week.

> *Better a meal with vegetables where there is love than a fattened calf with hatred (Proverbs 15:17)*

5. Use a salad sized plate for your meals. If it does not fit, do not force it. No "sky high" piles either.

You do not have to be perfect in your nutrition habits. Any change you make towards healthier eating is an accomplishment. Neither do you have to completely eliminate foods you love to eat. Moderation and balance are key!

A balanced nutrition plan for average person ≈

Fat: 20-30% of total calories
Protein: 10-35%
Carbohydrates: 45-65%

Food And Faith

———ᗌᏉᏉ———

"If you do not change your direction, you may end up
where you are heading."—Lao Tzu

Where are you headed? Where are your daily decisions, habits
and thoughts leading you? Where do you want to go? Will your
current decisions, habits and thoughts get you there? Think about
these questions and be honest in your self-assessment.

*A truthful witness gives honest testimony, but a false witness tells
lies (Proverbs 12:17).*
Ask these very same questions as it relates to your nutrition.
Will your current lifestyle (nutrition, exercise, etc.) choices get you
to the state of health you wish to attain? If you answered yes, then
CONGRATULATIONS! Keep up the good work. But if you are
like many of us, including myself, the answer is no and your choices
are a work in progress.
You first have to change the way you think about food, and you
can do that by reading and practicing God's Word.
*My son, pay attention to what I say; listen closely to my words.
Do not let them out of your sight, keep them within your heart for
they are life to those who find them and health to a man's whole body.
(Proverbs 4:20-22).*
We can all change our actions briefly to suit the need of the
moment. But if you do not change the thought process behind
those new and improved patterns, you will inevitably fall back into
the same detrimental routine. Know the reasons why your actions
need to change both physically and spiritually. You want to change
your actions, so physically the body can be healthy, perform its
duties efficiently and effectively and improve your function in your

day-to-day activities, as well as your productivity in advancing God's kingdom. You want to change your actions spiritually, so you can glorify God.

So whether you eat or drink, or whatever you do, do it all for the glory of God (1 Corinthians 10:31).

Use this scripture throughout your journey to help guide your eating habits. You may say, "How can I glorify God with my eating habits?" Well, you can in several ways. You can do so by eating foods that will preserve your body, God's temple. You can be an example for your family and those around you, thereby helping to preserve God's people. And lastly, eating healthier improves brain function, therefore making you more receptive to retaining God's Word. Not to mention that a healthier you is better able to perform God's will. If you know that a particular food, beverage or habit you choose is going to harm your body, the temple of the Holy Spirit, would that be glorifying God?

Begin changing the way you think about food by praying for guidance.

Ask, and it will be given to you; seek, and you will find; knock, and the door will be opened to you. For everyone who asks receives; he who seeks finds; and to him who knocks, the door will be opened (Matthew 7:7–8)

Food is for nourishment and sustenance. Of course it can be enjoyed, but should not be used for a significant source of pleasure and/or comfort; it is a means to fuel the body. The next time you eat, ask yourself these questions:

1. Why Am I Eating This?
2. Do I just enjoy eating it?
3. Am I trying to mask my pain and it comforts me?
4. Am I hungry and need to replenish?
5. Will this help me glorify God?

If you answered yes to number 3, you may be using food to satisfy a void in your life. You may use food to comfort in times of pain, fill emptiness, suppress anger, satisfy a need or simply to fulfill any inner longing you may have. Your hunger pangs may be an indication that your soul is starving.

Man shall not live by bread alone, but by every word that proceedeth out of the mouth of God" (Matthew 4:4)

We fill our stomachs instead of filling the emptiness in our spirit and taking the time to deal with the real issues we are having. You may be dealing with the death of a loved one, low self-esteem, a broken heart, family disruptions, etc. One of the easiest ways to cope is to smother those feelings with food. That is why fasting can be a great tool; you no longer have the immediate gratification from food and can focus on figuring out your real issues, and rely on God to fill you up, comfort and satisfy you.

Praise be to God and Father of our Lord Jesus Christ, the Father of compassion and the God of all comfort, who comforts us in all our troubles . . . (2 Corinthians 1:3-4)

My soul will be satisfied as with the richest of foods. (Psalm 63:5)

Ask God for clarity in the midst of your situation and know that he can satisfy all your needs and fill any voids or longings you may have.

And my God will meet all your needs according to his glorious riches in Christ Jesus (Philippians 4:21)

You cannot eat your way out of your situation. You can devour any and all the food you want, but when you are done that emptiness still exists.

But food does not bring us near to God (1 Corinthians 8:8)

Just as with any other substance, food can be abused. In cases of alcohol abuse or drug abuse, you remove the substance from your presence and abstain; you have a resolution. But no one can abstain from food. Therefore mastering your eating habits is an ongoing process. You have to eat to live, and not falling back into the same pattern is hard-work.

Re-evaluate what you are eating, why you are eating it and when. If you are not hungry and do not feel the need to refuel, try putting off your eating until you are. Change what you are eating. If the item you chose will not help improve or maintain your health, then choose another item you like that is much healthier for you.

No long-term habit is going to change overnight. It takes time. So persevere and let God lead you and use you to glorify his name.

Prayer

———❦———

Father God, I submit my mind, thoughts, will and emotions to you.
I choose to align myself with your word.
Please guide me in your way, so that my thoughts and decisions line
up with your Word.
Thank you for filling me with your Holy Spirit and guiding me as I
take great care in trying to preserve your temple.
Thank you for empowering me to live the life of victory you have
in store for me.
Victory in my health, my nutritional habits and overall well being.
Victory in all my doings that glorify your name.

AMEN

Establishing Your RMR

―――― ⌒⌒ ――――

Your resting metabolic rate (RMR) represents the minimum amount of energy required to keep your body functioning, or to sustain life in a resting individual. Essentially, it is the amount of energy (measured in calories) used by the body to remain in bed asleep all day. RMR is responsible for burning up to 70% of the total calories used, but this figure can vary due to different factors (see below). RMR is the largest factor in determining overall metabolism and how many calories a person needs to maintain, lose, or gain weight.

These different factors are:

1. Genetics: some people are born with faster metabolisms and some with slower ones.
2. Gender: Men have a greater muscle mass and a lower body fat percentage. This means they have a higher RMR.
3. Age: RMR reduces with age. After age 20, it drops about 2% per decade.
4. Weight: The heavier the weight, the higher your RMR is. For example: the metabolic rate of an obese woman is 25% higher than that of a thinner woman.
5. Body Fat Percentage: The lower a person's body fat percentage, the higher the RMR. The lower body fat percentage in men is one reason why men have a 10-15% faster RMR than women.
6. Exercise: Exercise not only affects body weight by burning calories, it also helps raise your RMR by building muscle.

Listed below is an equation for calculating your RMR. It can be used to give you an estimate of your metabolic rate, but be advised that this equation does not take into consideration muscle mass, which can increase RMR measurement.

Harris–Benedict Formula To Calculate Your Metabolic Rate (RMR)

Women:
655 + (4.35 x weight in pounds) + (4.7 x height in inches) – (4.7 x age in years)

Men:
66 + (6.23 x weight in pounds) + (12.7 x height in inches) – (6.8 x age in years)

Because the equation does not take into account body composition (a measure of the percentage of muscle mass and fat mass of your body), it is less accurate if you have a non-typical amount of muscle. Muscle burns more calories because it takes more energy to sustain than fat.

A person with an above average amount of muscle will have a higher RMR than calculated; a person with a below average amount of muscle will have a lower RMR than calculated.

As you age, your RMR decreases because of a decrease in muscle mass and hormone production. When your weight goes down, your RMR goes down as well. If you have less body mass to maintain, then your body does not need as many calories to keep it functioning. This means that as you get older and lose weight, your RMR will decrease and you will need to eat less or exercise more to maintain your current weight.

Calculate your current RMR using the Equation to get an estimate of your daily caloric needs. Place that information below.

Calculate Your Metabolic Rate (RMR)

Women:
655 + (4.35 x weight in pounds) + (4.7 x height in inches) - (4.7 x age in years)

Men:
66 + (6.23 x weight in pounds) + (12.7 x height in inches) - (6.8 x age in years)

My RMR = _____ calories/day

Counting Calories

———— ⌇ ————

To lose, maintain or gain weight, learning basic knowledge about calories and how they work is necessary. A calorie is a unit of energy-producing potential that is contained in food and used in the body to produce energy. Calories are used to fuel our daily activities as well as exercise. To achieve weight loss, gain or maintenance, you must be able to estimate the calories you consume (take in) and burn off per day. It is all about "Calories In vs. Calories Out". If your goal is to lose weight, you want to consume less calories than you burn off. To maintain your weight, your calorie consumption and expenditure need to be the same. To gain weight, you would have to eat more calories than you burn off.

To understand how many calories your body burns, you need to establish your Resting Metabolic Rate (RMR). Your resting metabolic rate (RMR) is the amount of calories you would burn at rest in a 24 hour period. If your RMR is 1500 calories and you consumed 1500 calories a day, you would not gain nor lose weight but maintain it.

RMR is very important because it establishes the baseline from which your caloric expenditure and consumption should be measured. To lose weight you must have a caloric deficit, where you consume less calories than you burn off. The body burns calories naturally through its daily functions of living that keep the heart pumping, breathing, digestion, etc., but you can burn more calories by exercising and adding activity into your daily routine.

Example:

Anne has a goal to lose two pounds per week. She currently weighs 200 pounds, and her RMR is 2000 calories per day. A pound is equal to 3500 calories. For Anne to lose two pounds in one week, she must have a caloric deficit of 7000 calories. To create this deficit, Anne can either consume fewer calories than her 2000 calorie RMR, get active and burn the calories, or a combination of both. A combination of both managing calories and shedding calories through increased activity is recommended.

> 1 Pound = 3500 calories
> 2 pounds = 2 x 3500 calories = 7000 calories
> Anne needs to have a caloric deficit of 1000 calories per day to reach her goal of two pounds/week. 7 days x 1000 calories = 7000 calories

This can be done by:

- Decreasing her caloric consumption by 1000 calories per day, which would only leave her with 1000 calories a day for eating. This significant decrease in food intake would be very difficult to maintain because she would most likely be hungry and have cravings throughout the day.
- Exercising and burning off 1000 calories/day. For most people, this is approximately two hours or more of steady aerobic exercise every day of the week, which would also be very difficult to maintain.
- Decreasing her calorie intake by 500 calories per day and also increasing her activity level to burn another 500 calories per day. Activity can include a combination of dedicated exercise and regular daily activities, such as taking the stairs at work and walking for 20-30 minutes.

Estimating the number of calories you consume daily is essential to reaching your goal weight. After all, how will the "calories in, calories out" weight loss formula work if you have no idea how many calories you eat every day? Because the average person does not measure or weigh their food, knowing what a portion size looks like will play a pivotal role in estimating your calorie consumption.

A portion size tells you how many ounces, grams, etc . . . are in one serving of food. Everything from your fruits and veggies to your meats has a specific portion size. Once you have established how many portions you are eating, you can calculate your calories by adding up the calories based on portion size.

1 gram carbohydrate = 4 calories
1 gram of protein = 4 calories
1 gram of fat = 9 calories

Portion Control

———— ⌘ ————

If you eat out at restaurants or live by the old adage, "clean your plate", you are probably eating more than you should. Many of us tend to underestimate the amount of food we eat and overestimate the recommended portion sizes for many foods. For example, try pouring out your usual portion of cereal and measure it. Then compare it to the portion size listed on the label. Chances are you are eating two or three times the amount on the label, which means you have doubled or tripled the amount of calories you thought you were taking in. Relating portion sizes to everyday items is an easy way to visualize what a true portion size really looks like, and will get you on the fast track to eating properly portioned meals.

Take a look at the recommended serving sizes on the USDA MyPyramid Food Guidance System. Get out a measuring cup or a food scale and practice measuring some of your favorite foods onto a plate so that you can see how much (or how little!) a serving is. This will help you "eyeball" a reasonable serving.

The following page, The Faith-FULL Portion Control Guide, contains pictures for better visualization of what a portion size should look like. You will also find the "Faith-FULL Portion Controlled Plate". It depicts what food groups your plate should contain when you prepare your meal.

To take the guess work out of eating healthfully, two sample meal plans have been provided, as well as a guide to aid you in reading food labels while you shop for groceries. While both meal plans provide the same amount of macronutrients (carbohydrates, proteins and fats), meal plan two is divided into five smaller meals per day, versus the four meals per day found in meal plan one. This smaller spacing in between meals helps increase your metabolism and stave off hunger.

Choose a meal plan that works best for you, or consult your local dietetic professional for a more individualized plan.

Faith -FULL Portion Size Guide

When eating healthy, knowing how much you consume is key. Often we misjudge the amounts of food we actually take in. Using the Faith Full Portion Size Guide will give you easy comparisons so you can take the headache out of judging a serving size.

1 Serving of <u>Vegetables</u> ≈ 1 cup

1 Serving of <u>Fruit</u> ≈ 1/2 cup

1 Serving of <u>Meat /Fish</u> ≈ 3 oz

1 Serving of <u>Fats/Oils</u> ≈ 1 tablespoon

<u>Grains/Starchy Vegetable:</u>

1 Serving of *Cereal* ≈ 1 cup

1 Serving of *Rice or Pasta* ≈ 1/2 cup

1 Serving of *Bread* ≈ 1 Slice

<u>Dairy:</u>

1 Serving of *Milk* ≈ 1 cup

1 Serving of *Cheese* ≈ 1 1/2oz.

1 Serving of *Yogurt* ≈ 1 cup

1 serving of *Ice Cream* ≈ 1/2 cup

Sweets

Reference each package food label

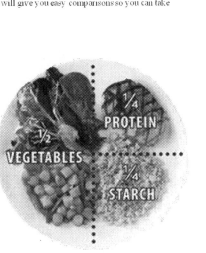

Baseball = 1 cup

Light Bulb = 1/2 cup

Deck of Cards = 3 oz Meat

Checkbook = 3 oz of Fish

Silver Dollar = 1 tbsp

3 Dice = 1 1/2 oz. of Cheese

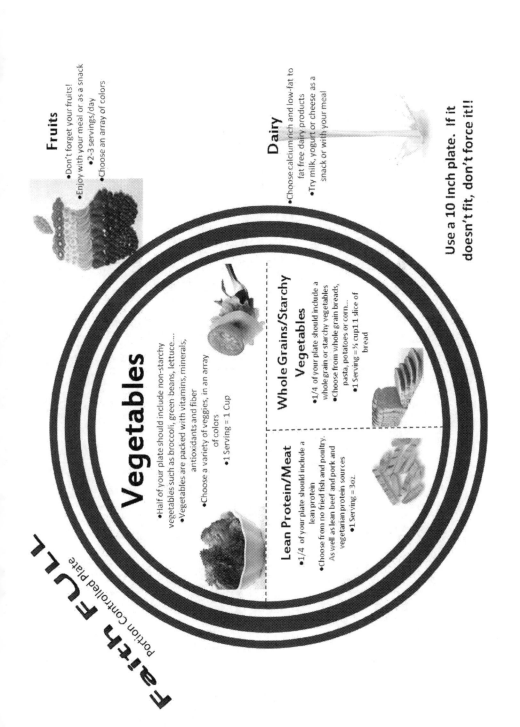

Faith FULL
Portion Controlled plate

Fruits
- Don't forget your fruits!
- Enjoy with your meal or as a snack
  - 2-3 servings/day
  - Choose an array of colors

Dairy
- Choose calcium rich and low-fat to fat free dairy products
  - Try milk, yogurt or cheese as a snack or with your meal

Use a 10 inch plate. If it doesn't fit, don't force it!!

Vegetables
- Half of your plate should include non-starchy vegetables such as broccoli, green beans, lettuce....
- Vegetables are packed with vitamins, minerals, antioxidants and fiber
  - Choose a variety of veggies, in an array of colors
    - 1 Serving = 1 Cup

Whole Grains/Starchy Vegetables
- 1/4 of your plate should include a whole grain or starchy vegetables
- Choose from whole grain breads, pasta, potatoes or corn...
  - 1 Serving = ¾ cup 1 slice of bread

Lean Protein/Meat
- 1/4 of your plate should include a lean protein
- Choose from no fried fish and poultry. As well as lean beef and pork and vegetarian protein sources
  - 1 Serving = 3oz.

Faithfully FULL Meal Plan One

Four meals a day (large breakfast, medium lunch, snack, small dinner)

<table>
<tr><th>THE PLAN</th><th>EXAMPLE</th></tr>
<tr>
<td>

Breakfast:
Drink at least 16oz. of water
2 Lean proteins
1 Fruit
1 Whole grain

Lunch:
Drink at least 16oz. of water
1 Lean protein
2 Veggies
1 whole grain

Snack:
Drink at least 16oz. of water
1 Fruit or veggie
1 serving lean protein
Or
Choose between a veggie, whole grain or fruit

Dinner:
Drink at least 16oz. of water
1 Lean protein
2 veggies
1 Whole grain

</td>
<td>

Breakfast:
Drink at least 16oz. of water
2 Eggs (remove one yolk)
1 Turkey sausage link or patty
1 banana
1 slice whole grain toast

Lunch:
Drink at least 16oz. of water
2 cups romaine lettuce salad
• (add other veggies you like)
• 3 oz grilled lemon pepper shrimp
• 1–2 tbsp of red wine vinegar for dressing
• ½ whole grain pita bread

Snack:
Drink at least 16oz. of water
1 cup of grapes
1 cup of Greek Yogurt
Or
Celery and carrots

Dinner:
Drink at least 16oz. of water
3oz Cajun seared chicken breast
½ cup red beans
½ cup rice
1 cup collard greens

</td>
</tr>
</table>

"Eat breakfast like a king, lunch like a prince, and dinner like a peasant."

Watch your portions!

Faithfully FULL Meal Plan Two

Five meals a day (meals are equally sized)

THE PLAN	EXAMPLE
Breakfast: Drink at least 16oz. of water 1 Lean protein 1 Fruit 1 Whole grain	**Breakfast:** Drink at least 16oz. of water 2 Eggs (remove one yolk) 1/2c strawberries 1 cup of oatmeal
Snack: Drink at least 16oz. of water 1 Fruit or veggie 1 serving lean protein	**Snack:** Drink at least 16oz. of water 1 apple and 24 almonds or 8 celery sticks and peanut butter
Lunch: Drink at least 16oz. of water 1 Lean protein 2 Veggies	**Lunch:** Drink at least 16oz. of water 3 oz grilled chicken breast 4 oz sweet potato 1 cup green beans
Snack: Drink at least 16oz. of water Choose between a veggie, whole grain or fruit	**Snack:** Drink at least 16oz. of water Small (1 cup) romaine lettuce salad w/ tomatoes 2 tbsp of balsamic vinaigrette for dressing
Dinner: Drink at least 16oz. of water 1 Lean protein 2 veggies 1 Whole grain	**Dinner:** Drink at least 16oz. of water 4oz grilled tilapia 1 cup steamed broccoli ½ cup wild rice

Drink at least half your body weight in ounces of water per day!

Watch your portions!

Feeding The Spirit Instead

———— ↝ ————

Eating any and everything shows a major lack of discipline and does not honor God. Over indulgence and laziness, whether in eating or other areas, are both issues that result from lack of self-control.

Like a city whose walls are broken down is a man who lacks self-control (Proverbs 25:28)

You can have many external rewards in place to keep you from over indulging, such as paying a dollar every time you eat something unhealthy, or treating yourself on the weekend for having a good nutritional week. But without self-control, these methods are useless. Self control is chosen and cannot be enforced by outside influences. Paul says that he "beat" his body into submission, which translates into him being in control of his body. Exercise and eating right shows self-control and does not allow the body to give in to every whim and craving.

Therefore I do not run like a man running aimlessly; I do not fight like a man beating the air. No, I beat my body and make it my slave . . . (1 Corinthians 9:26)

Do not join those who drink too much wine or gorge themselves on meat . . . (Proverbs 23:20)

Do not be gluttonous in your eating habits. It can have adverse consequences and negatively affect your health long term.

. . . Is not life more important than food . . . (Matthew 6:25)

When you have eaten your fair share of food and you still have hunger pangs, feed your spirit. God can quench your thirst and satisfy your hunger,

For he satisfies the thirsty and fills the hungry with good things (Psalm 107:9)

Quench your excessive thirst and hunger with God's Word, because you are most likely trying to feed emptiness within.

. . . I have treasured the words of his mouth more than my daily bread (Job 23:12)

His Words can satisfy more than any of the richest foods. Blessed are those who hunger and thirst for the righteous Word of God. It is not the sustenance of this world, but Jesus who is your bread of life.,

Then Jesus declared, I am the bread of life. He who comes to me will never go hungry, and he who believes in me will never be thirsty (John 6:35).

There is no food richer and more fulfilling than God's Word.

. . . Listen, listen to me and eat what is good, and your soul will delight in the richest of fare. (Isaiah 55:2).

The Bible says, eat what is good and your soul will be satisfied just as if you ate the most tempting foods. God will fulfill you.

My soul will be satisfied as with the richest of foods (Psalm 63:5).

Therefore, fill your spirit and not your belly.

Some of us may see food as a constant temptation and it is an ongoing battle to refrain from eating too much. No one wants to gorge themselves on food, only to later regret it. Your mind wants to do one thing, yet you find yourself doing another.

I do not understand what I do, For what I want to do I do not do, but what I hate I do (Romans 7:15).

But that too can be overcome with God.

No temptation has seized you except what is common to man. And God is faithful; he will not let you be tempted beyond what you can bear. But when you are tempted, he will also provide a way out so that you can stand up under it. (1 Corinthians 10:13).

No temptation is greater than God. Not food, drugs, sex or any other—none!

You are not alone, for everyone has been tempted in some way. He will not put more on you than you can bear. Nor will He leave you to fight this battle alone. He will give you a way out! You just have to follow His lead.

As stated before in the Food and Faith chapter, food should not be used as your source of fulfillment, but as sustenance for the body. Food is a gift from God for which we should be thankful, and that gift should never be abused. Heather Harpman Kopp says in *The Dieter's Prayer Book* that "Ultimately every source of food is a gift, a provision from God's hand. And when we adopt this attitude of gratitude, we actually defuse food's power over us. Think of it this way; we do not abuse what we're thankful for. We abuse what we're angry at ourselves for wanting in the first place." So be thankful.

Prayer

———⌇———

Lord,
Increase my appetite for your Word and decrease
my appetite for external satisfaction.
Give me the strength to exude self control in the midst
of my temptations.
Feed my spirit, so that I may be satisfied.
You are my bread of life and you alone sustain me.
Lord, fulfill me, so I only crave the goodness of your love
Show me your way oh God and allow me to feast on you Lord,
that my spirit may be filled.
Thank you God for keeping me and providing me
with all that I need.

AMEN

Grocery Shopping

—◌◌—

Did you know there is an art to grocery shopping? No . . . not really, but there are a few tips you should consider to help you make healthier choices while shopping.

The very first thing you want to do prior to your trip to the grocery store is assess what food items you already have and what food items you need. Compile a list and write out the needed items, grouping them so items that are in the same area of the store are listed together. Once you have assessed your needs, revise your list according to items that fit within your nutritional plans. All other items should be eliminated from the list or replaced with healthier options. Creating a grocery list prior to shopping and sticking to that list will help you save money, and help you make healthier, more thought out food choices.

Now you are ready to head to the store. Remember to park as far away from the door as possible and burn a few extra calories!. When shopping, try to get most of your foods from the outer ring of the grocery store. This is where most of your fresh food products are located, as well as your fresh fruits, dairy, whole grains, lean meats and vegetables. Most of your processed foods are located down the center aisles. Although all processed foods are not bad, you want to limit the amount you take in. Aim for fresh food, rather than manufactured food products.

Be wise in your food choices. If it is questionable then try to find a healthier option. Remember moderation and balance are key—you do not have to cut out everything you enjoy. If you want to eat your favorite dessert, you may have to eat fewer calories at your next meal. "The key to weight loss is cutting fat and calories where it hurts the least," says Connie Diekman RD. "Eliminate calories from your nutritional plan where you will not miss it as much. Do not sacrifice the foods you love. Doing so will only increase your desire for them. Instead, eat smaller portions and eat them less often." Choose seasonings with low to no sodium amounts, such as garlic powder (not garlic salt), black pepper and herbs. Opt for beverages that are low in sugar. You can also pick natural juices for your flavored beverages, such as orange, grape or apple juice. Just be mindful of the portion sizes you use and the calories you are taking in. You do not want to blow a tremendous amount of your daily calories on beverages. Choose high fiber and whole grain breads, cereal and pasta.

All items in the store other than your fresh vegetables, fruits and meats will have food labels. READ the LABEL carefully for serving size, calories and nutrients. This will give you an indication of whether that particular product will work well within your nutritional regimen. Use the food label guide and quiz on the following pages to help you understand how to read a food label.

Following the section on food labels are lists of healthy foods broken down in categories of vegetables, fruits, whole grains, lean meats, seasonings, sweeteners and beverages. You can take the lists with you to the grocery store to aid you in making healthier food choices. Or you may choose to make your grocery list from each category prior to your trip.

Understanding Food Labels

———— ⌒⋄ ————

Become a smart shopper by reading food labels to find out more about the foods you consume. The nutrition facts panel found on most food labels will help you find out:

- How many servings are in the container?
- How many calories are in each serving and the entire package?
- What nutrients does the product contain, such as fiber, calcium, iron, and vitamin C?
- How many grams of protein, carbohydrate and fat are in the product?

Begin with the Serving Size

Look for both the serving size (the amount for one serving) and the number of servings in the package. Remember to check your "actual" portion size to the serving size listed on the label. If the serving size is one cup and you eat two cups, you are getting twice the calories, fat and other nutrients listed on the label.

Assess the Total Calories and Fat

Find out how many calories are in a single serving and the number of calories from fat. It is a wise choice to cut back on calories and fat if you are watching your weight.

Use the Percent Daily Values

Use percent Daily Values (DV) to help you evaluate how a particular food fits into your daily meal plan. Daily Values (DV) are the average amounts of nutrients for a person eating 2,000 calories a day. Percent DV are for the entire day, not just for one meal or snack. You may need more or less than 2,000 calories per day. Use your calculated RMR (resting metabolic rate) to assess your caloric needs.

Your Goal

Aim low in total fat, saturated fat, trans-fats, cholesterol, and sodium; 5% or less for each is considered low. Aim high in vitamins, minerals and fiber. 20% or more is considered high.

Nutrition Facts

Serving Size 1 Cup (228g)
Servings Per Container 2 — Start Here

Amount Per Serving

Calories 250	Fat Calories 110	Check the calories

		% Daily Value*	
Total Fat	12g	18%	%DV Quick Guide
Saturated Fat	3g	15%	5% or less is low
Trans Fat	3g		20% or more is high
Cholesterol	30mg	10%	
Sodium	450mg	20%	Limit these
Total Carbohydrates	31g	10%	
Dietary Fiber	0g	0%	Get adequate amounts of these
Sugars	5g		
Protein	5g		

Vitamin A	5%
Vitamin C	3%
Calcium	25%
Iron	0%

* Percent daily values are based on a 2,00 calorie diet. Your daily values may be higher or lower depending upon your calorie needs

Using guidelines on reading food labels, answer the following questions pertaining to the food label on the previous page.

1. How many servings are in this container? _____
2. How many calories per serving? _____
3. How many calories would you consume if you ate the entire container? _____
4. How many grams of fat are there? _____ How many grams of saturated fat are there? _____
5. How many grams of carbohydrates? _____
6. How many grams of protein? _____
7. Calculate the calories of carbohydrates, proteins and total fat in this container.

1 gram carbohydrate = 4 calories
1 gram of protein = 4 calories
1 gram of fat = 9 calories

_____ calories of carbohydrates
_____ calories of protein
_____ calories of fats

Answers: **1.** two **2.** 250 **3.** 500 **4.** 12g fat, 3g saturated fat **5.** 31g **6.** 5g **7.** 31x4=124 carbs, 5x4=20 protein, 12x9=108 fats

Vegetables

——— ✤ ———

Vegetables should be a constant staple in any diet. The benefits they offer are well documented. Vegetables contain essential vitamins, minerals, and fiber that may help protect you from many chronic diseases. Eating vegetables is a great way to make a poor diet healthier and get many of the nutrients you need to stay well.

Every vegetable is not included on this list. But all vegetables are good for you. So choose any!! Try fresh, frozen or low sodium canned vegetables with fresh and frozen being the best choice. Also using "steam in bag" vegetables and steam bags you can put in the microwave can reduce your cooking time if you have a hectic schedule.

VEGETABLES

Alfalfa Sprouts	Chives	Parsley
Artichoke	Collard Greens	Peppers
Artichoke Hearts	Corn	Potato (white or red)
Arugula	Cucumber	Pumpkin
Asparagus	Eggplant	Radicchio
Avocado	Endive	Radishes
Bamboo Shoots	Green Beans	Rhubarb
Bean Sprouts	Green Onions	Rutabaga
Beets	Green Peas	Sauerkraut
Bell Peppers	Greens	Shallot
Black Eyed Peas	Horseradish	Snow Peas
Bok Choy	Jicama	Soy Beans
Broccoflower	Kale	Spinach
Broccoli	Kohlrabi	Split Peas
Cabbage	Leeks	Summer Squash
Carrots	Lemon Grass	Sweet Potato/Yam
Cauliflower	Lettuce (various)	Tomato (various)
Celery	Lima Beans	Turnip Greens
Chard	Mushrooms	Water chestnuts
Chickpeas	Mustard Greens	Watercress
Chile Peppers	Okra	Winter Squash
Chinese Cabbage	Onions	Zucchini

Fruits

———— ✺ ————

Fruits are one of the best sources of carbohydrates you can choose. Carbohydrates are sometimes measured by the effect they have on the body's blood sugar levels. This measure is called the **Glycemic Index (GI)**. Carbohydrates that break down quickly during digestion and release glucose (sugar) rapidly into the bloodstream have a high GI. Carbohydrates that break down more slowly, releasing glucose more gradually into the bloodstream, have a low to medium GI. For diabetics, choose carbohydrates with a low to medium GI to keep blood sugar levels balanced. Foods with adequate amounts of fiber usually have a lower GI.

Fiber is the indigestible portion of plant foods (vegetables, whole grains and fruits), and is essential to proper digestion. It works in the intestine to help remove waste from the body.

Women need ≈20 grams of fiber a day
Men need ≈30 grams of fiber a day

If you are relatively healthy and diabetes is not an issue, the GI does not need to be strictly adhered to, so you may enjoy any fruits you would like.

FRUITS

LOW GI FRUITS	HIGH GI FRUITS	HIGH FIBER FRUITS
Cantaloupe	Watermelon	Bananas
Rhubarb	Any Dried fruit	Pears
	Blueberries	Apples
MEDIUM GI FRUITS	Figs	Strawberries
	Grapes	Oranges
Apples	Kumquats	Raspberries
Fresh Apricots	Logan Berries	Kiwi
Bananas	Mangos	Guavas
Blackberries	Mulberries	Avocado
Cherries	Pears	Figs
Cranberries	Pineapple	Blue Berries
Grapefruits	Pomegranate	Grapefruits
Guava	Prunes	Acai Berry
Kiwis		
Lemons		
Limes		
Oranges		
Papayas		
Peaches		
Plums		
Raspberries		
Strawberries		
Tangerines		
Tomato		

The Great Whole Grain Debate

Whole grains are grains that have not gone through the refining process, where they are stripped of their outer shell (bran and germ). During this process, grains lose much of their nutritive value and fiber. Whole grains offer more nutritive value than refined grains because they contain more fiber, vitamins, and minerals (such as potassium and magnesium). Studies have shown that taking in adequate amounts of whole grains can reduce your risk of heart disease, prevent some types of cancer and help with weight loss as well.

Many products claim to be whole grain but only possess trace amounts of whole grains. True "whole grain" products will be made mostly of whole grains and limited amounts of refined grains. When in doubt about choosing the best product, check the label. Look for the word "whole" on the package, and make sure whole grains appear among the first items in the ingredient list. Also, try to choose items with at least 3 grams of dietary fiber per serving.

Choosing whole grain bread can be tricky. Brown bread does not equal whole grain. Look to see if the bread has whole seeds still intact. Multi-grain does not equal whole grain. This label simply means different varieties of grains are in the product. Look for products that list the number of whole grains in grams. For 1-2 servings, eight grams would be a good source; sixteen grams indicates an excellent choice. Look for products that list the percentages of whole grains. A 100% whole grain label would be your top choice.

WHOLE GRAINS

Whole grains:	Refined grains:

Whole grains:

Brown rice
Buckwheat
Bulgur (cracked wheat)
Oatmeal
Popcorn
Barley
Granola

Ready-to-eat breakfast cereals:

Whole wheat cereal flakes
Muesli
Whole grain barley
Whole grain cornmeal
Whole rye
Whole wheat bread
Whole wheat crackers
Whole wheat pasta
Whole wheat sandwich buns and rolls
Whole wheat tortillas
Whole wheat pitas
Whole wheat bagels
Whole wheat or rye flour
Wild rice

Less common whole grains:

Amaranth
Millet
Quinoa
Sorghum
Triticale

Refined grains:

Cornbread★
Corn tortillas★
Couscous★
Crackers★
Flour tortillas★
Grits
Noodles★
Pasta★
Spaghetti
Macaroni
Pitas★
Pretzels

Ready-to-eat breakfast cereals

Corn flakes
White bread
White sandwich buns and rolls
White rice
White flour

★ Most of these products are made from refined grains. Some are made from whole grains. Check the ingredient list for the words "whole grain" or "whole wheat" to decide if they are made from a whole grain. Some foods are made from a mixture of whole and refined grains.

Some grain products contain significant amounts of bran. Bran provides fiber, which is important for health. However, products with added bran or bran alone (e.g., oat bran) are not necessarily whole grain products.

Lists were compiled by the USDA and can be found: **http://www. mypyramid.gov/pyramid/grains.html**

Proteins

———— ෴ ————

Proteins provide the building blocks of muscle and are vital to enzyme and hormone production in the body. Proteins help you stay satisfied longer and are essential in a balanced nutrition plan. Proteins can be found in all meat, but not all protein has to come from animal sources. Vegetables, beans and grains can be great supply of protein as well. Although most non-animal sources of protein are incomplete proteins (do not contain all 9 essential amino acids), combining various vegetables, legumes or grains in one meal or throughout the day can supply you with the 9 essential amino acids the body needs. For example, combining beans and rice will give you the nutrients found in a "complete" source of protein.

Faith-FULL and Fit lists various animal proteins by the fat content they contain, ranking them from very lean to medium fat proteins. Vegetarian protein sources are listed thereafter.

VERY LEAN	LEAN	MEDIUM FAT
= 35 calories, 1gram fat/oz	= 55 calories, 2-3gram fat/oz	= Proteins 75 calories, 5gram fat/oz
Chicken breast-no skin	Salmon	Whole egg
Turkey breast-no skin	Turkey Dark Meat—no skin	Mozzarella cheese
Venison (deer meat)	Chicken Dark Meat—no skin	Pork Chop - No noticeable fat
Bison (buffalo)	Herring	Ricotta Cheese (1/4cup)
Fish Fillet -tilapia, flounder, sole, scrod, cod, bass, whiting, etc…	Swordfish	Tofu (4oz)
Shellfish-clams, lobster, crab, scallop, shrimp	Lean Beef - flank steak, London broil, tenderloin, roast beef	
Cottage cheese - non/low fat	Sardines	
Egg whites	Veal - roast or lean chop	
Egg substitute	Lamb - Roast or lean chop	
Fat Free Milk or cheese	Fresh ham	
Beans-cooked black beans, kidney, chick peas or lentils	Pork tenderloin	
Soy	Low Fat Milk and Cheeses (3gm of fat or less/oz.)	
	Low fat luncheon meats (3gm of fat or less/oz.)	
	Cottage cheese	

*1 serving = 3 ounces

VEGETABLE PROTEIN

Artichokes
Beets
Broccoli
Brussels sprouts
Cabbage
Cauliflower
Cucumbers Eggplant
Green peas
Green pepper
Kale
Lettuce
Mushrooms
Mustard greens
Onions
Potatoes
Spinach Tomatoes
Turnip greens
Watercress
Yams
Zucchini

GRAINS

Amaranth
Barley
Brown rice
Buckwheat
Millet
Oats
Oatmeal
Quinoa
Rye
Wheat bran
Wheat germ Wheat
Wild rice

LEGUMES

Adzuki beans
Bengal gram
Black beans
Broad beans (fava)
Chickpeas
Cowpeas (catjang)
Falafel
French beans
(mature seeds)
Garbanzo beans
Hummus
Kidney beans
Lentils
Lima beans
Miso
Moth beans
Mung beans
Mungo beans
Navy Beans
Pigeon peas
Pink beans
Pinto beans
Soybeans
Split peas
White beans
Winged beans
Yardlong beans
Yellow beans

FRUIT PROTEINS

Apple
Banana Cantaloupe
Grape
Grapefruit
Honeydew melon
Orange
Papaya
Peach
Pear
Pineapple
Strawberry
Tangerine
Watermelon

OTHER SOURCES OF PROTEIN

Tofu
Soy Products
Veggie burgers
Meat substitutes
Nuts
Whey
Casein
Veggie protein
powders

Beverages

———— ༄ ————

Beverages are any liquid you consume by mouth other than water. Items such as juice, soda and milk are considered beverages.

What is a caloric beverage? Any liquid you consume that has calories in it, e.g., juice, soda and sweet tea.

When drinking caloric beverages, use a 4oz–8oz cup! Once that is gone, quench your thirst with water. Be mindful of how many ounces of caloric beverages you consume. The calories can add up quickly and will hinder your progress if you're not keeping track. They add to your daily caloric count just as food does. So limit your consumption of caloric beverages and use water as your main source to alleviate your thirst.

Avoid high sugar beverages (other than those with natural sugar) like punch, juice cocktails, juice-flavored beverages, sweet tea or anything you add extra sugar to for enhanced flavor.

LOWEST CALORIE*	GOOD CALORIC BEVERAGES*
Water (add lemon, ginger, vanilla, orange slices, mint or cucumber)	Vegetable Juices
Herbal Tea	Apple Juice
Coffee (no sugar)	Pomegranate Juice
Diet Soda	Prune Juice
Low-calorie flavored water	Grape Juice
Low-calorie electrolyte beverages	Tomato Juice
Low-calorie flavored drink packages	Grapefruit Juice
	Cherry Juice
	Acai Berry
	Cranberry Juice
	Orange Juice
	Including but not limited to the above

*   *Based on caloric content and nutritive value*

Seasonings And Herbs

———— ❧ ————

Herbs and spices are a great, easy way to add flavor to your food without adding sodium (salt). You know what you like better than anybody, so why not make your own seasonings? It is just a matter of trial and error. You combine seasonings when you cook all the time, so just put it in a jar. Save an old seasoning shaker and remove the label. Choose your favorite low-sodium seasonings (<35mg/serving), combine them in a bowl, place it in your shaker and presto! You have the best low sodium seasoning in town.

Try these combinations:

- Mexican Blend: cilantro, garlic powder, black pepper and crushed red pepper

- Italian Blend: minced onion, minced garlic, black pepper and Italian seasoning

Use one of the following, or blend a few together and make your own.

Dried Herb Blends	Garlic Powder	Black Pepper
Jerk Seasoning	Basil	Oregano
Rosemary	Thyme	Lemon Grass
Chicory	Mustard	Chives
Dill	Cumin	Nutmeg
Bay Leaves	Caraway	Celery Seed
Cardamom	Cayenne Pepper	Cinnamon
All Spice	Ginger	Tamarind
Tarragon	Turmeric	Vanilla
Chile Pepper	Cilantro	Sage
Sassafras	Saffron	Cloves
Coriander	Curry	Fennel
Horseradish	Capers	Sesame
Parsley	Water Cress	Cilantro
Mint	Licorice	Parsley
Italian Seasoning	Red Pepper	Lemon

Reducing Your Sodium (Salt) Intake

———— ᴄⱴꙅ ————

Sodium is a mineral. The main dietary source of sodium is common table salt (sodium chloride), but regular unprocessed foods contain natural sodium as well. Sodium is sometimes used as preservatives to inhibit the growth of food-borne pathogens (especially in luncheon meats, fermented foods, salad dressings, and cheese products). Sodium, when over-consumed, can cause issues such as high blood pressure and weight gain. According to the American Heart Association, you can limit your sodium consumption in the following ways.

- Cook your own foods. When you cook your own foods, you know what seasoning it is prepared with.
- Choose fresh, frozen or canned food items without added salts.
- Select unsalted nuts or seeds, dried beans, peas and lentils.
- Limit salty snacks like chips and pretzels.
- Avoid adding salt to homemade dishes.
- Select unsalted, lower sodium, fat-free broths, bouillons or soups.
- Learn to use spices and herbs to enhance the taste of your food. Most spices naturally contain very small amounts of sodium.
- Add fresh lemon juice instead of salt to fish and vegetables.
- Specify how you want your food prepared when dining out. Ask for your dish to be prepared without salt.
- Do not use the salt shaker. Use the pepper shaker instead.

According to the USDA, **healthy adults** should have **no more than 2,400mg** (or about one tsp) of sodium a day in their entire nutritional plan.

A daily **limit of 1,500 mg of sodium** (<3/4tsp) is generally considered a healthy, low sodium diet plan. This plan is good for individuals with high blood pressure.

SODIUM EQUIVALENTS

¼ Teaspoon Salt" 600mg of Sodium
½ Teaspoon of Salt: 1200mg of Sodium
¾ Teaspoon of Salt: 1800mg of Sodium
1 Teaspoon of Salt: 2400mg of Sodium

Sodium free:	Less than 5 milligrams of sodium per serving
Very low sodium:	35 milligrams or less per serving
Low sodium:	140 milligrams or less per serving

Sweeteners

———— ⌐⌐ ————

We all love our sweet desserts and beverages. But taking in too much sugar can have adverse effects on our health. So the next time you have a craving for sweets, try using natural and artificial sweeteners instead of processed sugar. Natural sweeteners come from nature and have not been chemically processed or altered. If you do not care for sweeteners, start by decreasing your sugar intake slowly. Reduce sugary foods and the amount of table sugar used. Remember, sugar can be found in baked goods, beverages, snacks and many of your everyday foods. Calories from sugar can add up quickly!

1 teaspoon of sugar = 15 calories

Even when substituting with sweeteners, be mindful of how much you use. Listed below are natural and artificial sweeteners that can be used as sugar substitutes. Remember to consider moderation with sweeteners as well.

NATURAL SWEETENERS	ARTIFICIAL SWEETENERS
Honey	Saccharin
Maple Syrup	Aspartame
Frozen Juice Concentrates	Sucralose
Stevia	Neotame—new form of aspartame without phenylalanine
Sucanat (sugar cane juice)	
Molasses	Sugar Alcohols (mostly in no sugar or reduced sugar foods)
Date Sugar	Prior to choosing an artificial sweetener, do your research. Read up on the positives and negatives about the product and use the one that is best for you.
Agave Nectar	
Rice Syrup	
Sorghum Syrup	

Cooked To Perfection

You have gone to the store and made some great selections and healthy choices. But when cooking your healthy food items, you do not want to add unnecessary calories by frying, adding excess amounts sugar, or adding fatty items like butter, buttermilk and fatback to enhance the flavor. Here are some healthy ways to prepare your food without adding extra calories.

- Bake
- Boil
- Broil
- Grill
- Poach
- Sear
- Sautee w/ Olive oil or cooking spray
- Steam
- Crock Pot
- Rotisserie
- Oven Fried

On the following pages are a list of common ingredients used in cooking to add flavor and texture. Next to them are healthy substitutions to keep the flavor but cut down on calories.

Faithfully Tasty Ingredient Substitution List

Now that you've stocked your cabinets and pantry with healthy foods, cooking healthier versions of your favorite recipes will be a snap. We have all had our share of "healthfully" revised recipes that taste like cardboard. However, modifying your favorite recipes so that they fit within your nutritional plan and keep the flavor is easier than you think. Try these healthier ingredient alternatives the next time you cook your family's favorite recipe.

RECIPE CALLS FOR:	SUBSTITUTIONS
SUGAR	
Sugar	Sugar substitute such as fruit juice concentrates, stevia and possible artificial sweeteners
Syrup	Pureed fruit such as applesauce, low-calorie or sugar free syrup
Fruit Flavored Yogurt	Plain yogurt with fresh fruit slices

RECIPE CALLS FOR:	SUBSTITUTIONS
FAT and CHOLESTEROL	
Butter, Margarine, Shortening or oil in baked foods	Try using half the amount called for or completely leave out if possible. Consider applesauce or other fruit purees.
Butter, Margarine, Shortening or oil to prevent sticking	Cooking spray or non stick pans
Salad Dressings	Reduced fat or fat free versions. Try salsa or flavored vinegars
Whole Milk/Evaporated Milk	Reduced fat or skim milk in regular and evaporated versions
Oil Based marinades	Fat free broth, cooking wines or fruit juices
Eggs	2 egg whites per one egg or egg substitute
Bacon	Turkey bacon, lean prosciutto or smoked turkey
Cream Cheese	Reduced fat or fat free cream cheese. Pureed fat free cottage cheese.
Sour cream	Reduced fat or fat free sour cream. Or plain yogurt
Mayonnaise	Reduced fat or fat free mayonnaise

RECIPE CALLS FOR:	SUBSTITUTIONS
SODIUM	
Any kind of salt; table salt, seasoning salt, garlic salt, etc..	Herb only seasonings such as garlic powder, pepper, minced onions
Soy Sauce	Low Sodium soy sauce
Preserved foods such as canned soups, sauces and frozen entrees	Prepare your own freshly made versions

RECIPE CALLS FOR:	SUBSTITUTIONS
LOW NUTRITIVE VALUE FOOD ITEM	
Chocolate	Dark chocolate or cocoa powder
White rice	Brown rice or wild rice
White flour	Whole wheat flour
Pasta	Whole wheat pasta
White bread	Whole grain bread. Whole grains should be listed as one of the top ingredients.
Iceberg Lettuce	Romaine lettuce, fresh spinach, arugula, mixed greens
Bread Crumbs	Bran flakes, rolled oats, almonds

Faithfully Full Eating Tips

———— ❧ ————

You have gotten your healthy foods and are cooking them to perfection. Use these helpful tips to go along with your healthy choices and cooking style.

Eat breakfast! Break your bad breakfast habits. You do not have to eat so-called "breakfast foods" for breakfast. You can eat anything that fits within the boundaries of your nutritional plan. Eating breakfast ignites your metabolism and prepares the body to start burning calories. So DO NOT SKIP it. It's true . . . breakfast is the most important meal of the day.

Drink a 16 ounce glass of water 20 minutes prior to a meal. It takes the brain 20 minutes to send a signal to the stomach that you are full and satisfied. Taking in water 20 minutes beforehand alerts the brain that you are eating and it prepares to send its "fullness" signal to the stomach. For the same reason, take at least 20 minutes to eat your meal. Eat slowly and enjoy your meal. This will give you time to converse with your family about the day's activities and events.

Choose one place in the house to eat. For example, only use the kitchen table. Whether it is a midnight snack or an evening meal, this is the only place you should eat. If you get fast food, wait until you get home to consume your meal if possible. This will help cut down on mindless snacking and add structure to your eating regimen.

Make sure your meals are portion controlled. If you want seconds and still feel hungry after your meal, drink 16 ounces of water, continue with your day's activities and wait 15 minutes. If your hunger has not subsided, choose one item from your meal to have seconds of, preferably the vegetables. Do not get seconds of everything and make sure whatever item you choose is portion controlled.

Fitness

———⚬⚬———

Physical training is good, but training for godliness is much better, promising benefits in this life and in the life to come (Timothy 4:8)

Beginning An Exercise Program

———⌒⌒———

Your body is the dwelling place of the Holy Spirit and should be taken care of.

"Do you not know that your body is a temple of the Holy Spirit, who is in you, whom you have received from God? You are not your own; you were bought at a price. Therefore honor God with your body" *(1 Corinthians 6:19-20).*

Praise God with your body by making it a healthy and welcoming place for God's Spirit to reside.

"After all, no one ever hated his own body, but he feeds and cares for it . . ." (Ephesians 5:29).

As with most things in life, there has to be balance; exercise is no different. You do not want to focus so much on your exercising that you neglect other areas of your life, and vice versa. Some people concentrate solely on their spirituality, to the neglect of their physical bodies. Others focus so much attention on the health and shape of their physical bodies, (exercise and nutrition) they overlook their spiritual needs and growth. Neither of these indicates a Biblical balance. First Timothy 4:8 tells us:

For physical training is of some value, but godliness has value for all things, holding promise for both the present life and the life to come

Note that the scripture does not exclude the need for exercise, and states that it is valuable. However, exercise has its place and the scripture prioritizes exercise accurately by saying that godliness is of superior value.

Healthiness and spirituality go hand and hand. To be in overall good health, one must not only be physically fit, but spiritually fit as well.

. . . I pray that you may enjoy good health and that all may go well with you, even as your soul is getting along well (3 John 1:2)

We must be spiritually fit and physically fit to do God's work and it is our duty to keep our bodies healthy and up to par.

There are many benefits to exercise. It can improve your body composition by helping you burn fat and improve muscular strength and tone. Exercise can increase your energy level, give you a euphoric feeling and reduce stress when certain hormones are released into the bloodstream during exertion. One of the greatest advantages to exercise is that it decreases the risk and prevents the onset of many diseases, such as diabetes, heart disease and obesity. But most importantly, it improves your overall health so you can concentrate on God's Word and perform his will for your life.

Exercise is a learned process and you have to teach the body what it should do by training it.

Like an athlete I punish my body, treating it roughly, training it to do what it should, not what it wants to . . . (1 Corinthians 9:27) TLB

You are what you repeatedly do. The activities you perform the most are the activities you perform the best. Therefore your exercising will be perfected with consistency and repetition. The same is true for your negative habits if they are what you do most often.

When starting an exercise program you should first consult your physician to make sure you are healthy enough to begin exercising. Make sure your fitness approach is well rounded and includes cardiovascular, resistance and flexibility training. Follow one simple principle: The F.I.T.T Principle.

> **F**—Frequency (3-5 Days per week). Frequency is the number of days per week necessary to achieve your goals.
>
> **I**—Intensity (60-85% of your maximum heart rate). Intensity is defined in relation to your maximum heart rate (for cardio exercises) and/or amount of weight used. It details how hard or easy your workout will be. Maximum heart rate can be calculated by subtracting your age from 220:
>
> 220—Age ≈ Max Heart rate

A 35-year-old person's max heart rate is 220-35 = 185.

T—Time (20 or more minutes each session). The amount of time spent doing continuous activity to achieve your goal.

T—Type is a specific exercise mode that will help you reach your goal. Choose any exercise that will keep your heart rate elevated (like walking biking, basketball, etc.) and that keeps your interest.

Remember to set goals. Begin by setting goals, both short term and long term. Make sure your goals are realistic, measurable and attainable. Set up a reward system for reaching those goals so you can enjoy your achievements.

Get an assessment of your current fitness level and design a program geared to improve the areas you need help on and maintain the areas that do not. Choose an exercise program that has activities that you enjoy! This is a must if you want to maintain your healthy activity program for a lifetime. Ask for help if you need it. Do not be afraid to ask what you may think is the simplest of questions.

Get a partner for added motivation. If you have someone to hold you accountable, you can help each other stick it out. Get your family involved. Not only will this help your family get healthy with you, it will bring you closer together.

Execute and refresh your program as needed. Once you feel as though your current exercise plan is getting too easy, challenge yourself and move to the next level.

F.I.T.T Principle

Choose Your Goal				
GOAL	**Frequency**	**Intensity**	**Time**	**Type**
Improve cardiovascular endurance. And aid in in increasing your daily tasks	At least 3 days per week	70 - 85% Max Heartrate or 7-8.5 on scale of 1-10 (How hard the exercise feels)	Warm-up for 3-5 minutes followed by 20 minutes of cardiovascular exercise in heart rate zone. Complete with 3-5 minute cool-down	Cardiovascular activity such as walking, biking, elliptical, jogging, etc..
Lower body fat	Aim for 3-5 days per week	65-70% Max Heartrate or 7-8.5 on scale of 1-10 (How hard the exercise feels)	Warm-up for 3-5 minutes followed by 30+ minutes of cardiovascular exercise. Complete with 3-5 minute cool-down	Cardiovascular activity such as walking, biking, elliptical, jogging, etc..
Improve muscle strength	2-3 Non-consecutive days per week	70% of your one rep max on a given exercise. Complete 2-3 sets of 8-12 reps	Rest for 2 minutes between sets	Machine circuit training, free weight exercises, body sculpting class
Improve muscle endurance	2-3 Non-consecutive days per week	2 or more sets, for 12-15+ repititions	Rest for 30-60 seconds between sets	Machine circuit training, free weight exercises, body sculpting class
Improve flexibility		Minimum of 2-3 days per week	Hold each stretch for 30-60 seconds	Stretch each major muscle group

- Note: Repetitions are guidelines. If 8-12 repetitions are recommended you should NOT be able to comfortably do 13!
- If you cannot do at least 6 or 7 your weight is most likely too heavy for regular weight training.
- When participating in Body Sculpting classes, be sure to use weight that is challenging but manageable.

★ *Guidelines based on those provided by the American College of Sports Medicine.*

Fitting Exercise Into Your Daily Routine

Sometimes jumping right into a new exercise program is neither convenient nor realistic. But you can begin by fitting exercise into your daily activities at home, in the office and on the go.

At Home

It is convenient, comfortable and safe to work out at home. It allows your children to see you being active, which sets a good example. You can combine exercise with other activities, such as watching TV and cleaning the house. Sometimes it is easier to have short bouts of activity several times throughout the day than it is to work out continuously for 30 minutes or more. Consider these tips provided by the American Heart Association:

- Do housework yourself instead of hiring someone else to do it.
- Work in the garden and/or mow the grass. Using a riding mower does not count!
- Rake leaves, prune, dig and pick up trash. You will be surprised at the calories you'll burn.
- Go out for a short walk before breakfast, after dinner or both! Start with 5-10 minutes and work up to 30 minutes.
- Walk or bike to the corner store instead of driving. When walking, pick up the pace from a leisurely stroll to a brisk walk. Choose a hilly route for added intensity.
- While watching your favorite show, sit up instead of lying on the sofa. And exercise during the commercial breaks.
- Stand while talking on the telephone.
- Walk the dog.

At the Office

With the advances in technology, many of our jobs are sedentary with little to no physical activity; even the need for walking down the hall to deliver a message has been eliminated with the advent of email and text messaging. Since, work takes up a significant part of the day, getting in even a little movement at work can be advantageous. Here are a few tips to add exercise in at work:

- Stand while talking on the telephone.
- Walk down the hall to deliver a message rather than using the telephone or email.
- Take the stairs instead of the elevator. If you are in a large building, get off the elevator a few floors prior to yours and take the stairs the rest of the way.
- When on business travel, stay at hotels with fitness centers and swimming pools so you can use them. Take along a jump rope and resistance band in your suitcase. Create your own indoor workout of cardio and band resistance training.
- Participate in or start a recreation league at your company, such as softball or Frisbee. You will improve your fitness and promote company morale.
- Join the company fitness center or local gym near your job. Work out before or after work to avoid rush-hour traffic, or drop in for a lunchtime workout.
- Schedule exercise time on your business calendar and treat it as any other important appointment or meeting.
- Get off the bus a few blocks early and walk the rest of the way to work or home.
- Walk around your building for a break during the work day or during lunch.
- Sit on a stability ball 10 minutes out of each hour during your work. Sit erect to promote good posture and strengthen the abdominal and lower back muscles.

At Play and On the Go

Play and recreation are important for good health. Look for opportunities to be active and have fun at the same time. Bring in the family as well. Let them get fit and have fun with you.

- Plan family outings and vacations that include physical activity (hiking, backpacking, swimming, etc.).
- See the sights in new cities by walking, jogging or bicycling.
- Make regular dates with your spouse or a friend to enjoy your favorite physical activities.
- Play your favorite music while exercising; choose something that motivates you and gets you pumped up.
- Dance with someone or by yourself. Take dancing lessons. Hit the dance floor on fast numbers instead of slow ones and boogie to the beat.
- When golfing, walk instead of using the cart.
- Park farther away at the shopping mall and walk the extra distance.

Cardio Exercising At Home

Are you like many of us who are not quite comfortable exercising around other people? Or maybe one or a few days out of the week you are unable to make it the gym. It could be that you do not have a gym membership at all. Whatever your reason, it does not have to be your excuse. When you are just starting out, you can get a great workout in the comfort of your own home. Just remember to do your cardiovascular activity for a minimum of 20 minutes for beginners and up to one hour in duration for the advanced exerciser. Choose one activity from below or combine a few.

- Walk the Stairs—use the bottom step of the staircase and step up and down. Be sure to switch feet and lead with both left and right legs.
- Walk around the neighborhood
- Do a cardio-based DVD

- Dance to your favorite tunes
- Play with the kids
- Walk the dog
- Exercise during the commercial breaks while watching television:
  - Do jumping jacks, air jump rope, body weight resistant exercises like squats and lunges for the lower body and pushups for the upper body
  - Various Punches and Kicks: Jab, Cross, Upper Cut, Hook, Front kick, side kick, back kick

The Workouts

———— ✑ ————

When many of us think about exercising, we envision carving out at least an hour of our time each day to head to the gym. But that does not have to be the case. Exercising for health purposes can be done in spurts throughout the day, at home or in the office.

AT HOME WORKOUT: CARDIO-SCULPT

Equipment:
- Resistance Tube

The Routine:
Complete this circuit 1-3 times as you are able.

1. Pushups (modified on knees, on wall or regular): 10-20 reps
   Stationary or walking Lunges: 20-30 reps
   Jumping jacks: 30-60 seconds
2. Row with resistance band: 10-25 reps
   Squats with resistance band: 10-25 reps
   Stationary defensive slide: 30-60 seconds
3. Alternating abdominal leg lifts: 10-30 reps
   Back extension: 10-25 reps
   Plank: 2 reps at 10-30 seconds
4. Dips (on stairs, side of tub, step etc): 10-25 reps
   Squat jumps: 10-20 reps
   High knee lifts: 30 seconds–1min
5. Bicep curls with resistance band: 10-25 reps
   Ab twists (seated, lean back & twist from side to side): 20-40 reps

Plank – 2 x 10-30sec

Beginners should start with the lower number of repetitions and duration in time. For example: in the first circuit, you would complete 10 push-ups, 20 stationary lunges and 30 seconds of jumping jacks.

Cool-down and stretch.

"ABOUT THE HOUSE" WORKOUT

With this workout, there are no excuses as to why you cannot work out at home. This workout uses your basic household items to get your heart pumping and sweat dripping.

Equipment:
- Two 1-gallon or ½-gallon milk jugs filled with water (or filled to a level you are comfortable lifting)
- Broom or mop
- 2 unopened soda or juice cans
- Kitchen/dining room table chair
- Empty space in your home and a hallway
- Your favorite "Boogie" music

The Routine:
- Aerobic step touch: 1 minute
- Aerobic step hop (over broomstick): 1 minute
- Squats (hold 1-gallon jug between legs. Using a chair as your guide, Squat down and graze the seat of your chair on your descent.): 1 minute
- With a soda cans in each hand, complete 2 minutes of the following exercises:
  - Alternating jabs
  - Alternating upper cuts
  - Bob and weave with a cross punch
  - Jab with opposite leg knee lift (both sides)

- Jog up the hallway then back pedal back to where you started: 1 minute. Follow with 10 pushups (any way you choose) after each minute. Complete 5 minutes
- Take your two 1 gallon or ½ gallon jugs and perform lunges with bicep curls: 1 minute
- Overhead triceps press: 1 minute
- Run in place (get those knees up):1 minute
- Air jump rope: 1 minute
- Toe touch crunches for 1 minute
- Scissor legs for 1 Minute

Repeat the circuit however many times you can in 30-60 minutes, depending on the length of your day's workout. Cool-down and stretch.

THE OFFICE WORKOUT

I hear you!! You do not have time in your day to do a structured workout. Who said it had to be structured. Every little bit helps.

THE TO DO LIST:

- Take the stairs everywhere you go. The elevators are off limits. Try to pretend like you live in the Stone Age and all the modern luxuries of today that keep us from moving our feet no longer exist.
- Invest in a stability ball. For ten minutes every hour, sit on this ball instead of your desk chair. No slouching backs!! Stay erect and keep those abdominal muscles pulled in tight. You will improve your posture and strength levels in your abdominals and lower back.
- If there is an errand that needs to be run, jump at the chance to get up out your seat.
- When coming in to work, park at the top level of the parking deck. You can either take the stairs or walk the ramps to get

to your destination. Repeat on your way back to your car in the evening.

- While at your desk, do 100 C-Curves. Sitting straight up, you will pull in and squeeze the abdominal muscles as tightly as possible until the body forms a semi "C".
- In your desk chair, perform knee lifts. Sit straight in your chair and lift one knee at a time to your chest. Increase your speed to get the heart rate up.
- Desk Hip Flexions: Sit up straight and lift both legs up with the legs extended out in front of you. You may alternate legs if you need to modify. This is a great abdominal workout.

Now you have the tools to work out during your day, without setting foot outside the office . . . . THERE ARE NO MORE EXCUSES. Getting healthy is only a work day away!

Stretching And Flexibility

Although often overlooked, stretching and acquiring flexibility play a big role in rounding out your exercise routine. Stretching helps reduce your risk of muscle injury, improves flexibility, joint range of motion and circulation. It can also aid in stress reduction.

A good stretching routine stretches all the major muscle groups for 20 seconds or more. Pictured below are a few stretching exercises you can use to build your routine.

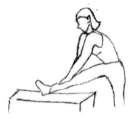

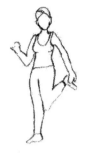

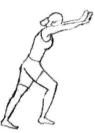

| Hamstring (Back of thigh) Stretch | Quadricep (Front of thigh) Stretch | Standing Calf (Back of Lower Leg) Stretch |

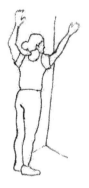

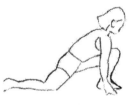

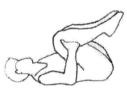

| Pectoralis (Chest) Stretch | Hip Flexor (Upper front of thigh) Stretch | Lumbar (Lower Back) Stretch |

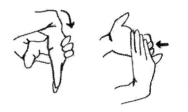

| Trunk (waist) Rotation Stretch |

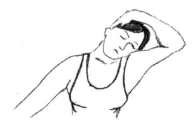

| Glute (butt) Stretch |

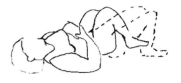

| Wrist Stretch |

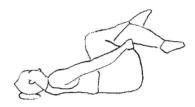

| Neck Stretch Stretch |

"I praise you because I am fearfully and wonderfully made; your works are wonderful, I know that full well"
Psalm 139:14

True Beauty And Happiness

---∽---

"You may not like me, but Jesus thinks I'm to die for!"

You are a beautiful and unique individual, made in God's likeness. Your mere presence is a blessing and you are truly a gift. You are loved effortlessly!!! And you are at your best just being you! With God as your guide, you will continue to be a blessing and be blessed.

That is how God sees you, fat or skinny, fit or out of shape. But I am sure there have been many times when you haven't felt beautiful, good enough or encouraged. Sometimes, life's tribulations can leave you battered, bruised and nothing but a shell of the person you once knew, often times leaving your self esteem on rock bottom and diminishing the glow that once surrounded you to nothing more than a dim shimmer. Life can sometimes cut so deep, you feel you have been left with scars that can never be removed. Yet, you are still a sight to behold!

How beautiful you are my darling. Oh, how beautiful . . ." (Song of Songs 1:15)

. . . Like a lily among thorns . . . (Song of Songs 2:2)

Society has taught us that beauty is the one who is sleek in stature with "awe"—inspiring features. We are considered beautiful when we receive admiring glances and are the envy of our peers. Do not be fooled by the world's definition of beauty, for it is vain and meaningless. True beauty lies within. You can have all the pretty packaging, but without a beautiful spirit, what are you really worth? Not much. After all, who just wants the wrapping paper and not the gift inside?

Your beauty should not come from outward adornment, such as braided hair and the wearing of gold jewelry and fine clothes. Instead, it should be that of your inner self, the unfading beauty of a gentle and quiet spirit, which is of great worth in God's sight (1 Peter 3:4)

Humble yourself like Christ. It is man that finds pleasure in your exterior appearance and accessories. Get your mind off man and get it on God, and you will see where your beauty truly lies.

Maybe you have tried to live up to the world's standard of beauty and fallen short. Too big, not pretty enough, too short, etc . . .

. . . He had no beauty or majesty to attract us to him, nothing in his appearance that we should desire him (Isaiah 53:2)

This is what they spoke of Jesus, yet he is the most beautiful person I know. Maybe your self esteem has been wrecked by people in your life that really did not have your best interest at heart. Let no one fool you into believing that you are not worthy and that they are better than you. We are all God's children—ALL have sinned and fallen short of his grace.

. . . If any one of you is without sin, let him be the first to throw a stone at her (John 8:7)

Even the one who is deemed as perfect, with the greatest praise has fallen short of God's glory. But we are ALL cleansed by his blood.

For God so loved the world that he gave his one and only Son, that whosoever believes in him shall not perish but have eternal life (John 3:16)

We are all saved by God's grace, not just the preacher, or those deemed to have the closest relationship with God

For it is by grace you have been saved, through faith . . . (Ephesians 2:8)

Through Jesus we are perfect and complete. Know who you are. You are chosen. You are the child of a King, an heir to salvation.

But you are a chosen people, a royal priesthood, a holy nation, a people belonging to God . . . (1 Peter 2:9)

Rebuild your self esteem knowing you are loved by God. He is able to look beyond your imperfections. A person who has God as the head of his life is the fairest of them all.

Charm is deceptive and beauty is fleeting; But a woman who fears the lord is to be praised (Proverbs 31:30)

Turn down the volume of your fears, your regrets and your resentments so you can hear from God. He says you are not defeated and you have nothing to be ashamed of. I have made you new.

Though your sins are like scarlet, they shall be white as snow; though they are red like crimson, they shall be like wool (Isaiah 1:18)

Do not listen to the fear-based advice your neighbors are so willing to give you. Do not let the negativity of the world discourage you and leave you feeling low.

Blessed are you when people insult you, persecute you and falsely say all kinds of evil against you . . . (Matthew 5:11)

Seek validation from God, not man. People will love you one day and not the next. Let God build you up instead of letting others tear you down with their inconsistencies.

It is better to trust in the LORD than to put confidence in man (Psalm 118:8 KJV)

Negative people are like black holes that seek to pull you in. When it seems that everything in your life is going wrong, something is going right. Look to God and be lifted.

Though my father and mother forsake me, the Lord will receive me. (Psalms 51:10)

God accepts you as you are, so accept yourself. Acceptance of self is essential to happiness and self love. Many people believe that all these worldly things—money, fame, external beauty—will make them happy. They pursue these ideals whole-heartedly, only to find the very happiness they so eagerly seek eludes them. That is because true happiness lies within the spirit. Jesus identified the key to happiness when he said: Happy are those that are conscious of their spiritual need.

Blessed are the poor in spirit, for theirs is the kingdom of heaven. (Matthew 5:3)

True happiness can only be found when you take steps to fill your greatest need, the hunger in your spirit. That hunger can only be fulfilled by being faithful to God's Word (The Bible), walking in his purpose for your life and believing in his unconditional love.

Let love and faithfulness never leave you; bind them on the tablet of your heart (Proverbs 3:3)

*"You are precious . . .
in my sight, and . . .
I love you"
Isaiah 43:4*

Knowing God's Word can help you discern what is important in life and what is not.

In all your ways acknowledge him, and he will make your path straight (Proverbs 3:6)

No more losing your "happy" over trivial non-sense. The petty things of the world fall to the wayside. Allowing God's Word to be your governor leads you to a more meaningful and fulfilling life.

. . . Blessed rather are those who hear the word of God and obey it. (Luke 11:28). Once you are filled in your spirit and realize where your true beauty lies, happiness will manifest and you can genuinely be accepting of yourself.

Prayer

————⌒⌒————

Lord transform my mind so that the world's idealistic view of beauty
is not my own.
Alleviate me of the shallow viewpoints I have adopted from society.
Yes, I want to be accepted and admired.
But teach me God that your admiration and acceptance is all I need.
Lord, touch me so that I may view myself as you see me.
Not as the world sees me, or even as I may see myself.
Press it upon my heart and engrave it upon my mind that I am a
Child of God.
Made like no other and I am unconditionally loved by you.
For there is no love greater than yours.
Open my eyes to see that my true beauty lies within and my
happiness resides in you.

AMEN

Free the spirit of its baggage,
And the body's baggage will
follow . . .
Carla T. Hardy

Losing Weight The Healthy Way

———— ❧ ————

We all want the quick fix and lose our extra pounds swiftly. Unfortunately, there is not one. Dropping weight too quickly can have adverse effects on the body and you are more likely to regain the pounds you have lost plus some if you do not step into change gradually.

When you make rapid changes, more often than not the methods you chose to get the weight off were unhealthy and were practices you could not sustain over a significant period of time, let alone a lifetime. After you dropped a few pounds, you probably fell back into your old routine.

To lose weight healthily, change your unfavorable habits little by little and replace them with healthy ones. Trying to change everything at once is a recipe for disappointment and failure. Remember the fable of the Tortoise and Hare? You want to be the tortoise in your pursuit of weight loss. Slow and steady wins the race and keeps the weight off. Small steps yield big results. Living healthy is a learned habit and, like any new task, it will take time to perfect. Have patience.

"But they who wait for the Lord shall renew their
strength; they shall mount up with wings like eagles; they
shall run and not be weary; they shall walk and not faint"
Isaiah 40:31

CONSISTENCY IS KEY

You should try to lose no more than 2-3 pounds per week. This is a healthy weight loss range to stay within. Stay consistent in your program and don't hop on and off the wagon. Just keep pushing!

Patience is a must. We are what we repeatedly do. Therefore, excellence is not an act, but a habit.

Do not be discouraged if your weight fluctuates day to day or throughout the day. Shifts in water weight, constipation, and even the food you just ate can cause the changes you see on the scale. These weight changes are particularly common during the beginning of a new healthy way of living, when your body is adjusting to your new eating habits. You may also notice that you weigh more immediately after a meal. This is due to the actual weight of the food and not to any fat weight you have gained. Remember that it takes time for your body to digest food and it can take a couple of days for weight loss or weight gain to register on the scale.

If you are trying to shed pounds, it is important to keep track of your weight. But can you ruin your motivation and success by weighing too often?

Weigh yourself at the same time and on the same scale for consistency. Weighing on various scales is a no-no! All scales are not equal and your weight may vary on each one. It is best to weigh in the morning just after you have awakened and have taken your morning bathroom break.

To avoid confusion and disappointment, weigh yourself only once a week or every other week. Let how much healthier you feel, your decrease in body fat percentage and how your clothes are fitting become your "scale" and measure for success.

Don't Give Up, Have Patience And Perservere

Take your time. What took years to create will not be broken down in a few short months, but will be an ongoing process of self renewal and encouragement. While the road to a healthy lifestyle may not be straight, it should not have many detours. You will have pitfalls and plateaus, but you should not totally go off path. Beginning and maintaining a lifelong healthy habit can be a struggle. Whether you are trying to lose weight, manage current disease states such as diabetes and high blood pressure, or continue on your healthy path, it will be a process. You must remember that you have to be patient. Just as your bad habits were solidified over a period of time, so will your new and improved ones.

. . . the race is not given to the swift or the battle to the strong . . ." *(Ecclesiastes 9:11).*

. . . but he who stands firm until the end . . . (Matthew 24:13).

Change your habits little by little. Remember, small steps yield big results. We are a society of quick fixes and want to see our results immediately. But all things come in God's time, not man's. Your blessing is on the way.

But if we hope for what we do not yet have, we wait for it patiently. *(Romans 8:25)*

Sometimes maintaining your motivation when you are not seeing the external results (such as weight loss on the scale) is hard. But pray for perseverance and strength to continue your journey.

. . . being strengthened with all power according to his glorious might so that you may have great endurance and patience . . . (Colossians 1:11)

If God has promised it to you, it will come in due time. Be encouraged and stay energized.

We do not want you to become lazy, but to imitate those through faith and patience inherit what has been promised (Hebrews 6:12)

Getting physically and spiritually fit the proper way will take much patience. And it may be difficult at times. What seems "hard" initially will become habit. The habit will become easy, and what's easy will become second nature.

"You need to persevere so that when you have done the will of God, you will receive what he has promised" (Hebrews 10:36).

You also have to have faith. Faith in God and faith in yourself and your abilities to finish what you started. Faith without works is dead.

" . . . faith without deeds is useless?" (James 2:20).

" . . . his faith and his actions were working together, and his faith was made complete by what he did" (James 2:22).

You have to do the work and know that the Lord will help manifest the results you desire.

There will be times when you want to give up and throw in the towel—when you have reached a plateau and the results are not coming as quickly as you would like, despite your valiant efforts. It is during these times that your faith in God is most valuable. You already know he will provide all your needs and desires, so why give up?

"Delight yourself in the Lord and he will give you the desires of your heart" (Psalm 37:4).

There will be times when you fall off the wagon and all the goals you want to accomplish are a distant memory; starting again seems like the hardest of feats. We have these setbacks not only in trying to improve our health but in life in general. We all fall short of God's glory. But with God, we all have the strength to get back up. Every day is a new start if you need it.

Therefore we do not lose heart. Though outwardly we are wasting away, yet inwardly we are being renewed day by day (2 Corinthians 4:16)

Sometimes you become a hindrance to your own progress. In these instances, you must hold yourself accountable for your actions. Really see your lifestyle and habits as they are. Whether it is poor nutritional habits or lack of activity, be accountable for them!

A truthful witness gives honest testimony, but a false witness tells lies. (Proverbs 12:17)

Be honest with yourself and begin to make small changes. Stop making excuses. "I am taking care of everyone else . . . But who is taking care of me??" "I am so busy, I do not have enough time in my day to get healthy." Well, make time! We always make time for the things we really want in life. Your physical and spiritual health is no different. If you are constantly making excuses as to why you cannot start or will not do this or that, then you are not ready for God's promises. When is your faith going to catch up with God's promise? Learn to love yourself enough and have faith enough to know that you do not need anyone but God to help you. He will not let you fail or fall.

When you have reached your breaking point and you feel as though your motivation to continue is nonexistent, be strong! Do not give up!

Have I not commanded you? Be strong and courageous. Do not be terrified, do not be discouraged, for the Lord your God will be with you wherever you go (Joshua 1:9)

To be blessed, you must first be broken and I am sure we all have been broken at some point in our lives. Once you have really been broken, you know beyond a shadow of a doubt that it was no one but God who was able to put your life back together.

I know what it is to be in need, and I know what it is to have plenty. I have learned the secret of being content in any and every situation, whether well fed or hungry, whether living in plenty or in want. I can do everything through him who gives me strength (Philippians 4:12–13)

If you feel as though you want to throw in the towel, I encourage you to hold on to your towel a little longer. You are going to need it to wipe away the tears of joy streaming from the blessings God is about to pour into your life! Do not give up on your goals, health related or otherwise. If God promised it to you, it shall be yours. Do not give up on God, because he will never give up on you. Just stand, because when there is nothing you can do, there is something God can do.

Prayer

———— ⌁ ————

Lord, please give me:

The strength to hold on
The courage to fight
The hope to pray
The faith to believe
The confidence to trust you
The patience to wait

Please renew my strength and my patience;
Help me to run this race of life and live for you
without becoming weary;
Although I may stumble
I know you will not let me fall.

AMEN

Faith

---⌒---

Doubt sees the obstacles, but faith
sees the way . . .
Anonymous

Your Faith-Full And Fit Plan

—— ✺ ——

Health and fitness is multi-faceted and requires a well-rounded approach. Decide which plan is going to work best for you and help you to reach your goals.

My Spiritual Plan—Keep God as the priority in your wellness plan. No matter what you are trying to do, God should be your guide. Any change on the outside begins on the inside. You are what you eat, drink, do and pray.

For as he thinketh in his heart, so he is (Proverbs 23:7) KJV

My Meal Plan—Choose your meal plan from the samples in the nutrition section of Faith-FULL and Fit, or follow one given to you by your physician/dietician if he/she has given you specific recommendations. Balance and moderation are key.

My Workout Plan—Choose a customized fitness workout that is geared to help you reach your goals. Do not just choose a plan because it worked for someone else. Consult your local fitness professional or choose one from the workouts plans provided within *Faith-FULL and Fit*. A complete workout plan will include cardiovascular, resistance and flexibility training.

Track your progress so you can see what you have accomplished. On the following pages you will find your *Faith-FULL and Fit* progress sheet to record your assessment results. Workout cards and food logs are also provided to track exercise and nutritional improvement. Your logs can also be used to make adjustments to your program if you are not reaping the results you desire.

Review your nutritional and exercise tracking if your results are less than desirable. Evaluate your exercise practices for consistency in your workouts. Also review your nutrition tracking to see if you are eating healthfully and your caloric intake is within the range set for your nutrition needs.

NAME:		DOB:		AGE:		HT.	
	INITIAL	2-WEEK	4-WEEK	6-WEEK	8-WEEK	10-WEEK	12-WEEK
DATE							

WEIGHT							
% Body Fat							

CIRCUMFERENCE MEASUREMENTS

SHOULDERS							
CHEST/BUST							
RIGHT ARM							
LEFT ARM							
WAIST							
HIP							
RIGHT THIGH							
LEFT THIGH							
RIGHT CALF							
LEFT CALF							

Faith Full Fit Workout Card

Resistance Training	Set #																													

Cardiovascular Exercises (Duration)

Cardiovascular workouts should be performed 3 to 5 times a week for a minimum of 20 minutes

Perform resistance training 2 to 3 times a week.
As a general rule, take at least a 30 to 60 second break between sets.
Remember to warm up and stretch before. And also cooldown after exercise training to help prevent soreness and increase flexibility.
Keep movements slow and controlled and use full range of motion.
Use variation in your workout program as it is the key to total physical conditioning.
Choose a variety of exercises for the entire body to improve total body conditioning.
Methods of increasing intensity: add more weight, increase sets, slow down movement or decrease rest time between sets

Target Heart Rate: _____ to _____ beats per minute   (Max HR = 220-age)   (Target Heart Rate = Max HR x .60 to Max HR x .85)

*Remember to warm up and cool down for at least 6-10 minutes.

Your Health Vs. Your Faith And Troubles

———— ⌀⅁ ————

When is your faith going to catch up with God's promise?

You have cried and cried. Depression has set in and you have begun emotionally eating and not exercising. Your peace is gone and staying healthy is the furthest thought from your mind. The worry lines have made a permanent home on your face. You have prayed and prayed. Yet you feel like your knocks on God's door have gone unanswered. While you are waiting on God, God is waiting on you. Yes, YOU!! He is waiting on you to have faith, concentrate and line up with his Word, change your thinking, and let go and let Him lead.

All the physical and spiritual changes you desire are within in your reach if you make glorifying God and bettering his kingdom your ultimate goal.

Have Faith

Have the faith of a mustard seed. Think about that. Could it be that you have not reached your goals because you have so little faith in your own abilities and in God to see you through?

Because you have so little faith. I tell you the truth, if you have faith as small as a mustard seed, you can say to this mountain, Move from here to there and it will move. Nothing will be impossible for you (Matthew 17:20)

If you do not have faith that you can attain the health and fitness goals you have set forth, you will never truly put in the effort it will take to reach them. No one would put 100% effort towards an outcome they feel they will never reach. Therefore you have to have faith.

Your faith is pleasing to God and it is impossible to please Him without it.

And without faith it is impossible to please God, because anyone who comes to him must believe that he exists and that he rewards those who earnestly seek him (Hebrews 11:6)

Whatever your pain, your stronghold, your affliction, your trouble, God is with you and he is able to bring change in your life. He can bring forth the change you desire in your health, your life circumstances and your spirit. You just have to have faith.

Build your spiritual foundation on your trust in God. You have to improve your kingdom thinking. Speak positivity into yourself. "I know that God is perfecting my life and my storm is only preparing me for what God has in store."

Our fathers disciplined us for a little while as they thought best; but God disciplines us for our good, that we may share in his holiness (Hebrews 12:10)

God will not give you blessings you are not yet ready to receive. You may be asking God for a better physique. But if God knows that you will not use it in a positive manner, he will not bless you with your desires until you are capable of doing so. He will not take you where your character will not sustain you. And your storms will do just that: build your character. Know that the trials you are going through are not for your destruction, but to get you to a place where God can bless you and give you the promises He already has in store for you. But you must walk by faith and not by sight.

Now faith is confidence in what we hope for and assurance about what we do not see . . . (Hebrews 11:1)

Although you cannot see it, believe it anyway. Your limited vision does not speak to God's power. Do not hinder yourself by focusing on what you can envision but have faith in God, because through Him all things are possible.

You want to lose weight but the mirror says you cannot. "You have always carried this weight and you always will." And you agreed. You want to be healthy but the doctor has given you a poor diagnosis. "Your disease state is out of control and there is no solution." And you believed him. Despite what you see, despite what you hear, you must have faith! Faith is the essential requirement and should be the foundation of your health and fitness regimen! You will see this come up time and time again. You start your fitness program and quit, or you are not seeing the results you want in a timely manner and you stop because you lack the faith that you will actually reach your goal. Most of our problems, in life and/or fitness stem from our lack of faith. If you know that God has it in his hands, then is there really a problem? If your faith is lacking, strengthen it by reading and exercising God's Word. Renew yourself through God's Word. Empower yourself with God's Word. God said I can quench your thirst eternally, not give you the temporary satisfaction found in man.

. . . Everyone who drinks this water will be thirsty again, but whoever drinks the water I give him will never thirst. Indeed, the water I give him will become in him a spring of water welling up to eternal life (John 4:13).

I will make rivers flow on barren heights, and springs within valleys. I will turn the desert into pool of water, and the parched ground into springs (Isaiah 41:18)

Trust in the Lord with all your heart and lean not on your own understanding (Proverbs 3:5).

Though your situation may seem bleak in your eyes, God has it all in control. The same God that delivered you before is the same God that will deliver you from your bad habits, strongholds and pain now. Pray.

Is anyone among you in trouble? Let him pray . . ." (James 5:13)

Depend on God for all things, including your health. If you believe that God is able and you trust him for your life, then there is no need to worry or doubt your goals and/or healing will come to pass. We all have problems, but the misery, stress, etc., come in when faith is not present and fear steps in. Your fear equals lack of faith, which leads you to worry over your situation. Your stress levels begin to increase, which in turn elevates blood pressure and increases weight gain. Weight gain invites obesity, and obesity brings along two best friends, diabetes and heart disease. Now your body's health is failing and riddled with problems, all because of your fear and lack of faith.

The enemy works through our fears, but God works through our faith. Faith allows us to see that our seemingly unreachable desires and goals will be met and brings peace in the midst of the storm.

Therefore, since we have been justified through faith, we have peace with God through our Lord Jesus Christ, through whom we have gained access by faith into this grace in which we now stand. And we rejoice in the hope of the glory of God. Not only so, but we also rejoice in our sufferings, because we know that suffering produces perseverance; perseverance, character; and character hope. And hope does not disappoint us, because God has poured out his love into our hearts by his Holy Spirit, whom he has given us (Romans 5:1-5)

Everyone has trials, the just and unjust alike.

A righteous man may have many troubles, but the Lord delivers them all (Psalm 34:19)

We all will have our season of storm at some point. If you never had a problem, you would never have the chance to exert your faith and give God the opportunity to solve them. Some of our troubles, we have brought upon ourselves. But lean on God anyhow; he can turn that around. God protects us even in the midst of our mess.

The Lord is close to the broken hearted and saves those who are crushed in spirit (Psalms 34:18)

Your faults and failures do not change God. He remains the same and His love is unconditional.

Jesus Christ is the same yesterday and today and forever (Hebrews 13:8).

You can be feeling low or walking the wrong path and God can still bless you right where you are. It is about the promise, not the environment or where you are in life. He has promised to supply your every need.

And my God will meet all your needs according to his glorious riches in Christ Jesus (Philippians 4:19)

More often than not our problems, heartaches and needs affect our health. They affect our drive to achieve better health as well. Therefore knowing how to deal with these circumstances when they surface in our lives is of utmost importance. Whatever your need, God has a promise for you.

In of need love:

If you are trying to get fit in order to receive love from man, you are doing it for the wrong reason. The shape of your body should not dictate the level of love a person has for you. God gives an unconditional love that no worldly love can compare to.

. . . I have loved you with an everlasting love; I have drawn you with loving-kindness. I will build you up again and you will be rebuilt (Jeremiah 31:3)

Know that if you love God, he will love you more.

No eye has seen, no ear has heard, no mind has conceived what God has prepared for those who love him (1 Corinthians 2:9)

And he is more faithful than any other.

Know therefore that the Lord your God is God; he is the faithful God, keeping his covenant of love to a thousand generations of those who love him and keep his commands (Deuteronomy 7:9)

God's love is unsurpassed and never falters as does man's love.

Though the mountains be shaken and the hills be removed, yet my unfailing love for you will not be shaken nor my covenant of peace be removed (Isaiah 54:10)

In need of financial prosperity:

Become a giver and not a taker. Acquire a giving spirit. No one gets blessed more than a giving soul.

Give and it will be given to you. A good measure, pressed down, shaken together and running over, will be poured into your lap" (Luke 6:38).

Stick with God. He says,

With me are riches and honor, enduring wealth and prosperity" (Proverbs 8:18).

A generous man will himself be blessed, for he shares his food with the poor (Proverbs 22:9)

Simply put, if you want to be blessed, be a blessing.

In need of joy:

Becoming fit will not give you joy. Yes, it will make you healthier and give you a nicer physique, but real, soul-stirring joy comes from God. You receive that joy by obeying God's commands. If your joy lies within the Lord, then man cannot take it away, no matter the situation.

I have told you this so that my joy may be in you and your joy may be complete (John 15:11)

Though you may me grieving or in poor health, there is still joy with God.

So with you; Now is your time of grief, but I will see you again and you will rejoice, and no one will take away your joy (John 16:22)

In need of healing:

Call on God and pray, then have faith that your healing will come to pass. If you pray and do not believe God will fulfill your need, you are praying in vain.

O Lord my God, I called to you for help and you healed me (Psalms 30:2)

Is any one of you sick? He should call the elders of the church to pray over him and anoint him with oil in the name of the Lord. And the prayer offered in faith will make the sick person well. The Lord will raise him up. If he has sinned, he will be forgiven. Therefore confess your sins that you may be healed. The prayer of a righteous man is powerful and effective (James 5:14–16)

In need of peace:

Seek to please God! Do so by having faith, praising and worshiping God even in the midst of your struggles. Remember that your praise and faith is pleasing to God.

When a man's ways are pleasing to the Lord, He makes even his enemies live at peace with him (Proverbs 16:7).

You will keep in perfect peace him whose mind is steadfast, because he trusts in you (Isaiah 26:3)

God's peace transcends all comprehension. His peace reaches depths that man will never understand.

And the peace of God, which transcends all understanding, will guard your hearts and your minds in Christ Jesus (Philippians 4:7)

There is no need to be worried or troubled. All you have to do is give your troubles to God.

Peace I leave with you, my peace I give you. I do not give to you as the world gives. Do not let your hearts be troubled and do not be afraid (John 14:27)

Go to Jesus with your burdens and lay them down at his feet.

Come to me, all you who are weary and burdened, and I will give you rest (Matthew 11:28)

In need of comfort:

Take solace in knowing that God sees your troubles and through him you will overcome. God is your strength, so lean upon him.

God is our refuge and strength, an ever present help in trouble (Psalm 46:1).

Though you may cry, He will wipe away every tear.

For the lamb at the center of the throne will be their shepherd; he will lead them to springs of living water. And God will wipe away every tear from, their eyes (Revelations 7:17).

In need of strength:

You are stronger than you think. If you have God, then you have all the strength you need.

He gives strength to the weary and increases the power of the weak (Isaiah 40:29)

The LORD gives strength to his people; the LORD blesses his people with peace (Psalm 29:11).

You are awesome, O God, in your sanctuary; the God of Israel gives power and strength to his people (Psalm 68:35)

In need of guidance:

First, you must stop trying to guide yourself. Let God lead you and light your path.

I will instruct you and teach you in the way you should go; I will counsel you and watch over you (Psalm 32:8)

I will lead the blind by ways they have not known, along unfamiliar paths I will guide them; I will turn the darkness into light before them and make the rough places smooth. These are the things I will do; I will not forsake them (Isaiah 42:16)

I have come into the world as a light, so that no one who believes in me should stay in darkness (John 12:46)

In need of health:

Exercise and proper nutrition can bring you physical health, but God gives spiritual health. What's on the inside manifests on the outside. Therefore seek to get spiritually healthy first. Fear the Lord and steer away from evil.

This will bring health to your body and nourishment to your bones (Proverbs 3:8)

Listen to and harbor God's word close to your heart.

My son, pay attention to what I say; listen closely to my words. Do not let them out of your sight, keep them within your heart; for they are life to those who find them and health to a man's whole body (Proverbs 4:20–22)

In need of protection:

The Lord will protect you always. If you keep God in your inner circle, there is no need to look any further.

The Lord will keep you from all harm—he will watch over your life; the Lord will watch over your coming and going both now and forevermore" (Psalm 121:7-8)

Regardless of the situation, God will keep you.

When you pass through the waters, I will be with you; and when you pass through the rivers, they will not sweep over you. When you walk through the fire, you will not be burned; the flames will not set you ablaze (Isaiah 43:2)

Looking for success:

We all want to feel that our hard-work is not in vain. We want to reach our goals and be successful in whatever we choose to do, whether in health or life. As long as God is your focus, you will always be successful. Recognize that all your successes come from him.

That everyone may eat and drink, and find satisfaction in all his toil—this is the gift of God (Ecclesiastes 3:13)

Moreover, when God gives any man wealth and possessions, and enables him to enjoy them, to accept his lot and be happy with his work—this is a gift of God (Ecclesiastes 5:19)

In need of mercy and forgiveness:

We have all made mistakes. God forgives you, and His mercy is upon you. Even when man cannot and will not forgive, God will.

Yet the Lord longs to be gracious to you; he rises to show you compassion. For the Lord is a God of justice. Blessed are all who wait for him! (Isaiah 30:18)

As a father has compassion on his children, so the Lord has compassion on those who fear him (Psalm 103:13)

In need of prayer:

Call on his holy name. The Lord hears and answers prayers.

This is the confidence we have in approaching God; that if we ask anything according to his will, he hears us (1 John 5:14)

The Lord listens, even when you feel He does not.

Then you will call upon me and come and pray to me, and I will listen to you (Jeremiah 29:12)

If you believe and have faith in God, then all these promises are yours. Faith gives you patience. There is no uncertainty with God, so do not doubt God. When you remove doubt from the equation, you give God the opportunity to do the impossible in your life. When you walk by faith, God will provide. The righteous shall live by faith and your faith is pleasing to God. Strengthen your faith from hearing and exercising God's Word.

You can choose faith, peace and good health. Or you can choose stress, worry and the inevitable demise in health that comes along with it. The choice is yours.

Concentrate and Line Up with God's Word

When you are going through times of trouble and sorrow, ask yourself, "are my actions in line with the Word of God?"

If you fully obey the Lord your God and carefully follow all his commands I give you today, the Lord your God will set you high above all the nations on earth. All these blessings will come upon you and accompany you if you obey the Lord your God (Deuteronomy 28:1-2)

Obey God's commands and you will receive blessings. Everything you need to ride out the waves of life can be found in your Bible. Read it and renew your strength. Read it and replenish your spirit. Read it and restore your health. People perish because of their lack of knowledge.

. . . my people are destroyed from lack of knowledge (Hosea 4:6)

But God will supply you with all the wisdom you need to navigate this world.

For the Lord gives wisdom, and from his mouth come knowledge and understanding (Proverbs 2:6).

. . . . He will teach us his ways, so that we may walk in his paths . . . . (Isaiah 2:3).

You cannot do what you do not know how to do. The guidance that you need and should seek is in God's word. Wisdom comes from God. He will provide you with all the knowledge you need to survive.

Many times we pray and ask God for things that do not line up with his will for our life, such as romantic partners who are not good for us, money and material things we do not need, sleek physiques to impress man, etc. What God has for you, is for you. And if it is in God's will, it shall be yours.

Now I commit you to God and to the word of his grace, which can build you up and give you an inheritance among all those who are sanctified (Acts 20:32)

So there is no need to worry or fret. While you are asking God for all these things, ask yourself, "Do my actions line up with God's will? Is this what God wants for me?" And be honest with yourself.

A truthful witness gives honest testimony, but a false witness tells lies (Proverbs 12:17)

If your answer is no, you now know and have insight as to why some of your prayers may have gone unanswered. The key is deciphering whether your desires are in line with God's will for you. You'll know your desires are in line if your desire is to build God's value and not your own.

Now if you ask yourself those questions and your actions do line up with God and your desires coincide with what God wants for you, you will get the desires of your heart.

Delight yourself in the LORD; and he will give you the desires of your heart (Psalms 37:4)

God wants you to live by his Word.

Fix these words of mine in your hearts and minds; tie them as symbols on your hands and bind them on your foreheads (Deuteronomy 11:18)

His Word is a light to your pathway. It should guide your day-to-day choices and be evident in your walk.

Your word is a lamp to my feet and a light for my path (Psalm 119:105)

Everything within the Bible is useful and can be used to shepherd you.

All scripture is God breathed and is useful for teaching, rebuking, correcting and training and righteousness. So that the man of God may be thoroughly equipped for every good work (2 Timothy 3:16)

Let God's Word become active in your day-to-day living and watch things change for you. Receive his knowledge and exercise it, just as you would anything else you want to become stronger and see growth in. You exercise your body on a consistent basis because you want to see changes in your health and shape. Exercise God's Word in the same manner, so you can see changes in your life.

Change Your Thinking

How do you view pitfalls, struggles and sorrow in your life? Do you think that God has somehow forgotten you? Or that life has let you down? You learn more and grow stronger from your failures and pain than you do from your successes. For example, you may have tried several fad diets and diet pills only to find that the promises on the package were not delivered. You may have been discouraged, but you learned that particular plan was not the best option for you.

Your troubles are not a negative entity to bring you down, as we have been often been taught they are, but a means to help you grow. For God is always with you, even in your darkest hours.

. . . Never will I leave you; never will I forsake you (Hebrews 13:5)

God wants you to change your thinking. View life's storms as positive and see what a difference it makes. You will find yourself no longer loathing your struggles, but gaining strength. If you continue to think negatively about your situation, you will find nothing but misery and depression. There are always two sides to every situation—choose the side that is going to build you up and not tear you down.

Finally, brothers, whatever is true, whatever is noble, whatever is right, whatever is pure, whatever is lovely, whatever is admirable—if anything is excellent or praiseworthy—think about such things (Philippians 4:8)

Positive energy begets positive energy. Positive doing begets positive doing in return. What you give out is what you receive in return. For example, it is by giving of yourself that you become rich. If you want to be rich, be a giver.

Turn your negative into a positive and get out of your own way. For instance: you may want to start exercising because you think you are too fat or do not like what you see in the mirror. Both of these attitudes stem from a negative view of yourself. However, if you change your motivation for exercise to a more positive reason, such as I want to be able to do more for the people in my life, you are more likely to stick with it. If you choose to look at everything positively, negativity is less likely to invade your space. If you are always unhappy and you cannot find peace with anything that you do, seek God. He does not wish that any of His children suffer needlessly and live without joy. God cares about all of us and would never bring what is wicked upon us.

. . . Far be it from God to do evil, from the Almighty to do wrong (Job 34:10)

God has a loving and great purpose for each of us.

Our fathers disciplined us for a little while as they thought best; but God disciplines us for our good, that we may share in his holiness. No discipline seems pleasant at the time, but painful. Later on however, it produces a harvest of righteousness and peace for those who have been trained by it (Hebrews 12:10-11)

We as humans see the test, but God sees the success. Do not concentrate on the struggle, but the victory you will gain once the battle has been won. Perceive troubles as a means for your personal and spiritual development in life.

My son, do not despise the Lord's discipline and do not resent his rebuke, because the Lord disciplines those he loves, as a father the son he delights in (Proverbs 3:11-12)

Nothing grows without rain. Coals cannot be made into a diamonds without a little pressure. Silver cannot be polished to a shiny new finish without some rubbing. We as humans are no different. We are perfected and transformed by our storms. You have to change the way you perceive life and troubles. You can change your actions briefly to suit the situation, but if you do not change the thought process behind your new actions, you are doomed to start making the same bad decisions. Think God's thoughts and you will receive God's results. What are God's thoughts? These are God's thoughts!

No, in all these things we are more than conquerors through him who loved us" (Romans 8:37).

. . . If God is for us, who can be against us (Romans 8:31)

I can do everything through him who give me strength (Philippians 4:13)

No weapon formed against you will prevail . . . (Isaiah 54:17)

In this life you may get burned pretty badly. But just like the phoenix, out of the ashes you will rise again, renewed and purified by the fire of God. Your pain has a purpose. There is no testimony without a test and no message without a mess. The way you perceive it all will determine the effect it will have on your life. Sometimes "it is not all about you". Your test may be the next man's blessing. They may find courage and hope for themselves in your testimony.

Give to others, and God will give to you. Indeed, you will receive a full measure, a generous helping, poured into your hands—all that you can hold. The measure you use for others is the one that god will use for you (Luke 6:38)

If you continue to think the way you have always thought, do you honestly believe you will receive different results? If you do what you have always done and think what you have always thought, you will get what you have always gotten. You have got to change your direction.

. . . but be transformed by the renewing of your mind (Romans 12:2)

You have to want to change. Sometimes we want God to do all the work. "If God wants me to leave it alone, he will take it away." "If God wants me to change, he will change me." "If God wants me to have it, he will give it to me." You have placed all the work on God. But you have to take some responsibility and do your part. You have to want to change for yourself. While you are waiting on God, he is waiting on you.

Without a changed mindset, you are spoiling your victory. You would not put fresh food into a contaminated container, for the fresh food would rot as well. The same goes for you. God cannot renew you with an unchanged mindset.

No one sews a patch of unshrunk cloth on an old garment, for the patch will pull away from the garment, making the tear worse. Neither do men pour new wine into old wineskins. If they do, the skins will burst, the wine will run out and the wineskins will be ruined. No, they pour new wine into new wineskins and both are preserved (Matthew 9:16-17)

Transform your thinking so old thoughts and patterns will die and leave room for God to do his work. But you first have to make the decision that you are ready to be renewed and the Holy Spirit will aid you in rest.

Let Go and Let God

Let God take the reins. He already has plans for you.

For I know the plans I have for you, declares the Lord, plans to prosper you and not harm you, plans to give you hope for a future (Jeremiah 29:11).

God can bring peace in the midst of your storm, so lay your cares at his feet.

Come to me, all you who are weary and burdened, and I will give you rest . . . (Matthew 11:28)

Realize and admit to yourself that your way is not working, whether it is in your daily life, or physical and spiritual health. There may be some things that God wants to add to your life, and some things he may want to remove. Let go and embrace the change he has set forth for you. "Let go and let God" is a phrase used often, but is sometimes easier said than done. But if you have faith, it is effortless. You may have the weight of the world on your shoulders—let it go. Let God carry that load for you.

Humble yourselves, therefore, under God's almighty hand, that he may lift you up in due time. Cast all your anxiety on him because he cares for you (1 Peter 5:6–7)

Footprints

One night a man had a dream. He dreamed he was walking along the beach with the LORD. Across the sky flashed scenes from his life. For each scene he noticed two sets of footprints in the sand—one belonging to him and the other to the LORD.

When the last scene of his life flashed before him, he looked back at the footprints in the sand. He noticed that many times along the path of his life, there was only one set of footprints. He also noticed that it happened at the very lowest and saddest times of his life.

This really bothered him and he questioned the LORD about it. "LORD, you said once I decided to follow you, you'd walk with me all the way. But I have noticed that during the most troublesome times in my life there is only one set of footprints. I don't understand why when I needed you most you would leave me."

The LORD replied, "My precious, precious child, I love you and I would never leave you! During your times of trial and suffering when you see only one set of footprints, it was then that I carried you."

Carolyn Carty, 1963

God is our refuge and strength, an ever-present help in times of trouble (Psalm 46:1)
Think back on your life and all the victories He has already brought you through, so you know that he is able. God can and will bring you through again. Maybe you are not out of your storm yet because you have been trying to navigate through it by yourself, with your flesh, in the physical.

The weapons we fight with are not weapons of the world. On the contrary, they have divine power to demolish strongholds (2 Corinthians 10:4)
You do not have to fight your battles alone. Fight with your prayer and your praise. Do not wait until your time of need to seek God. Praise him when things are good. Noah built his ark long before the storm came by doing as God commanded, and you should do the same.

Let your troubles go and have enough faith and belief to turn your situation over to God. Once you have handed it to God, worry no more and rest easy. Go to sleep knowing God has it under control and it has been taken care of. Your deliverance comes when you let it go. Both David (Psalms 3) and Peter (Acts 12) turned it over to God and worried no more. They rested because they knew that God would sustain them, even when they knew their lives were in danger.

I lie down and sleep; I wake again, because the Lord sustains me" (Psalms 3:5). "The night before Herod was to bring him to trial, Peter was sleeping between two soldiers . . . (Acts 12:6)
Stop trying to fight, fix and make it on your own. When your family and friends cannot help and you have tried it your way, try God's way. The battle is not yours to fight.

. . . 'Do not be afraid or discouraged . . . For the battle is not yours, but God's (2 Chronicles 20:15)

Cease trying to figure it out and let God work it out. Just because you do not have a remedy does not mean God is without one.

Even when God is working things out for our good, we may still need a little encouragement. When times get hard, encourage yourself.

The Twenty Third Psalms

The Lord is my shepherd; I shall not want. He maketh me to lie down in the green pastures, he leadeth me beside the still waters. He restoreth my soul; he leadeth in the paths of righteousness for his name's sake. Yea, though I walk through the valley of the shadow of death, I will fear no evil: for thou art with me; thy rod and thy staff comfort me. Thou preparest a table before me in the presence of mine enemies: thou anointest my head with oil; my cup runneth over. Surely goodness and mercy shall follow me all the days of my life: and I will dwell in the house of the Lord forever.

God has promised that all things work together for the good of those who love and serve him faithfully, including those situations you feel are unbearable.

And we know that in all things God works for the good of those who love him, who have been called according to his purpose (Romans 8:28)

It may be difficult for you to see and understand how God will bring this to pass in difficult times, but God has promised it, and he will deliver.

They that sow in tears, shall reap in joy (Psalm 126:5)

Everything you need to calm your storms can be found in your Bible and via knee-mail. Get your prayer on!

Prayer

———— ✎ ————

Dear God,

My light in darkness, my peace within the storm
Increase my faith and renew my thinking
Teach me your will and show me how to walk in it.
Lord, I know I have to endure this storm for my growth.
Lord you said that once I decided to follow you, you would walk
with me all the way.
Please God, change my thoughts on how I perceive this test.
Let me view my storm as a sign that I am progressing and you are
preparing me for my blessing.
Thank you for increasing my strength and polishing
my soul to a *lustrous* finish.
Help me to no longer see my troubles as a negative, but a means to
increase my faith and get closer to you oh Lord; to depend on you
for all my needs.
For I know that you will never leave nor forsake me.
Where I have doubt and worry God, replace with a renewed faith
that your word and love will see me through.
Father I stretch my hands to thee, in the midst of my storm, for I
know you are able.
Every tear I have cried, you wanted to wipe away
Every pain I have endured, you have wanted to erase
God I know you will make a way, just as you have done many times
throughout this storybook of my life.
I praise you Lord whether happy or sad, in joy or in sorrow.
You are my rock and my refuge
Thank you for loving me when I felt unloved and was
undeserving of your adoration
Thank you for all that you have done,
all that you are doing and will do.

AMEN

I Am Faith-Full And Fit

———— ⌁ ————

Dear friend, I hope all is well with you and that you are as healthy in body as you are strong in spirit (3 John 1:2) NLT

If you have reached the conclusion of this book, you have the basic knowledge you need to become spiritually and physically fit. They work hand in hand. As long as you have the Lord as your Shepherd to guide you through life's journeys, including health and fitness, you will reach your goals.

If you take away nothing else, take away this: Your faith is your greatest asset to your health and reaching your fitness goals. Remember that your body is the dwelling place for the Holy Spirit and should be treated and cared for as such. There will be times when it gets hard and the activities of life get you off track. But press your way and never give up, for God has promised you the desires of your heart.

Stay steadfast and active, for faith without works is dead. Though God will answer your prayers, some action is required on your part. Through it all, whether good or bad, progressing or reaching a plateau, keep the faith. God will bring you through this endeavor as he has done all others.

Now say it out loud! And profess to all . . .
I AM FAITH-FULL AND FIT!

Resources

———— ✿ ————

The New International Version Study Bible

King James Bible

New Living Translation Bible

Carla Hardy, MS, CSCS

Transcendent 360 Health and Fitness LLC

ACSM Guidelines for Exercise Testing and Prescription 8th Edition. 2009. Lippincott Williams & Wilkins

Clark, Nancy. 2008. Sports Nutrition Guidebook. 4th Edition. Human Kinetics

Harpham Kopp, Heather. 2005. The Dieter's Prayer Book (Spiritual Power and Daily Encouragement). Water Brook Books

Hafer, Tom P. 2006. Faith and Fitness (Diet and Exercise for a Better World). Ausburg Fortress.

Foster, Richard. 2002. Celebration of Discipline: The Path to Spiritual Growth. Zondervan Publishing.

www.about.com

www.eatingwell.com

www.fitfood.com

www.southernfood.com

www.hacres.com

www.americanprofile.com

www.cdkitchen.com

www.about.com

www.familyfun.com

www.medicinenet.com

www.cookinglight.com

www.southernliving.com

www.mealsmatter.org

www.mayoclinic.com

www.kraftfoods.com

www.familyfun.com

www.thatsmyhome.com

www.caloriesperhour.com

www.webmd.com www.aesm.org

www.byrdbaggett.com

www.theotherwhitemeat.com

www.helpguide.org

www.health.gov/dietaryguidelines

www.examiner.com/healthy-food-in-minneapolis/
helpful-hints-for-selecting-whole-grain-food

www.mypyramid.gov/pyramid/

www.appleseeds.org/100_Journaling.htm

www.nosaltnosugar.com

www.americanheart.org

www.dinewise.com

www.everydayhealth.com

www.care2.com

www.cfsan.fda.gov/label.html www.bmi-calculator.com

Printed in the United States
by Baker & Taylor Publisher Services